Fertility Treatment

In-Vitro Fertilization (IVF)

Akmal El-Mazny

CONTENTS

	PAGE
INTRODUCTION	1
DEFINITIONS	2
EVOLUTION OF IVF	4
INDICATIONS OF IVF	7
TECHNIQUE OF IVF	17
– PRE-CYCLE ASSESSMENT	17
– CONTROLLED OVARIAN HYPERSTIMULATION	24
– OOCYTE RETRIEVAL	39
– OOCYTE MATURATION	45
– SPERM PREPARATION	48
– INSEMINATION AND FERTILIZATION	52
– EMBRYO DEVELOPMENT	55
– EMBRYO TRANSFER	61
– POST-EMBRYO TRANSFER	66
RISKS OF IVF	69
– OVARIAN HYPERSTIMULATION SYNDROME	70
FACTORS AFFECTING IVF OUTCOME	82
IVF-RELATED TECHNIQUES	93
– INTRACYTOPLASMIC SPERM INJECTION (ICSI)	93
– GAMETE INTRAFALLOPIAN TRANSFER (GIFT)	97
– ZYGOTE INTRAFALLOPIAN TRANSFER (ZIFT)	99
– EMBRYO CRYOPRESERVATION	101
– ASSISTED HATCHING (AH)	108
– PREIMPLANTATION GENETIC DIAGNOSIS (PGD)	111
REFERENCES	116

INTRODUCTION

IVF is an assisted reproductive technology in which sperm and oocytes are retrieved and combined outside of the body where fertilization occurs, the embryos are then transferred to the uterus.

Initially developed for tubal factor infertility, IVF is now indicated in a broad range of situations and is very successful.

IVF is highly technological and has a number of rare though important risks, and must be used only after careful consideration of the medical indications and practitioners involved.

Multiple techniques are used to enable and improve IVF including intracytoplasmic sperm injection, embryo cryopreservation, assisted hatching, and preimplantation genetic diagnosis.

Hopefully this book will enhance your knowledge of IVF along with its appropriate indications and technique, and you will be able to apply this information to your professional practice.

DEFINITIONS

Assisted reproductive technologies (ARTs) are defined as all procedures in which oocytes and spermatozoa, or embryos are manipulated in-vitro for the purpose of establishing a pregnancy.

In-vitro, meaning in glass, describes procedures performed within a controlled laboratory environment rather than in vivo, or within a living organism.

In-vitro fertilization (IVF) is an ART in which sperm and eggs are retrieved and combined outside of the body in a laboratory dish where fertilization occurs.

The fertilized eggs or embryos are then transferred to the uterus with the hope one will implant and develop into a viable fetus.

IVF-Related Techniques

−Intracytoplasmic sperm injection (ICSI),

−Gamete intrafallopian transfer (GIFT),

−Zygote intrafallopian transfer (ZIFT),

−Gamete and embryo cryopreservation,

−Assisted hatching (AH), and

−Preimplantation genetic diagnosis (PGD).

IVF Terminology

– Prezygote is a fertilized pronuclear oocyte with male and female pronuclei.

– Zygote refers to a fertilized one-cell stage without nuclei, before cell cleavage.

– Preembryo is the conceptus during cleavage stages and until 14 days post-fertilization (when the primitive streak develops).

– Morula is the preembryonic stage from 16-cell to blastocyst formation (usually between 72 and 96 hours post-insemination).

– Blastocyst refers to the postmorula preembryonic stage in which a fluid-filled blastocele develops along with an inner cell mass.

– Embryo is the conceptus from primitive streak development until major organ development at the end of the 8th post-ovulatory week.

– Fetus is the conceptus from end of 8th post-ovulatory week until birth.

EVOLUTION OF IVF

Edwards and Steptoe first described the technique for IVF in 1976 and the subsequent births of two normal babies in 1978.

Since then, the success rate of the system has been improved (to 30%) by the use of fertility drugs to provide more oocytes and prematuration to mature the oocytes before fertilization.

The techniques of ART are now used in 53 countries throughout the world; in 1993, the results of 492 units from all over the world were collected from national surveys and registers.

Since 1985, more than 53,635 women had been treated and 34,316 babies had been born from 224,473 treatment cycles, following more than 160,518 transfer cycles.

Only about 65-75% of all resulting pregnancies attained live births; the remainder ended with spontaneous abortions (26%), or ectopic pregnancies (5.54%).

The multiple pregnancy rate (22%) was higher than the normal population and contributed to higher rates of preterm deliveries and perinatal mortality.

No increased incidence of chromosomal alterations and malformations were noted during the years (2.25%).

Since the birth of the first IVF baby, tremendous developments have occurred regarding the indications for ART.

For example, the dramatic development concerning male infertility which initially was considered to involve a small fraction of patients benefiting from IVF, now with the development of intracytoplasmic sperm injection (ICSI), involves up to 35% of started cycles.

Use of gonadotropin releasing hormone (GnRH) agonists has improved pregnancy rates, reduced blood sampling and prevented natural ovulation.

The disadvantages of stimulated cycles include higher risks of multiple pregnancy, hyperstimulation and side effects of the drugs.

Natural cycles or immature egg collection (IOC) may become alternatives to the use of the stimulated cycle.

Multiple pregnancies may be reduced, by reducing the number of eggs or embryos transferred.

Embryo freezing has made an important contribution to overall pregnancy rates by enabling patient to use excess eggs and embryos, the social and legal concerns resulting from the use of frozen embryos requires new ethical and legal consideration.

Micromanipulation of sperm and eggs has enabled fertilization and conception when sperm are defective in quantity and quality.

In summary, ART has developed over a decade to become useful for couples with infertility which cannot be cured by simple treatments.

The birth rates are comparable to natural conception and the incidence of congenital malformations is not increased.

The costs and complexities of treatment have been reduced, which in turn has reduced the stress and social inconvenience of therapy.

Problems related to the birth risk of multiple pregnancy and the use of the stimulated cycle are being reduced, as new techniques for severe male infertility and the detection of genetic abnormalities in the embryo have been introduced.

INDICATIONS OF IVF

Indications for IVF include mainly the bilateral absence or disease of fallopian tubes, and severe male factor infertility (defined as less than 5-10 million total motile sperm in ejaculate or surgically retrieved sperm).

Tubal Infertility

Tubal infertility is defined as persistent bilateral tubal obstruction, absence of tubes or tubal damage which has resulted in a period of infertility of more than 12 months' duration.

Possible therapy of tubal infertility includes hysterosalpingogram, chromatography at the time of laparoscopy, selective transcervical tubal cannulation and falloposcopy.

Each of their effects is restricted to the mechanical defect that may involve the tubal pathology.

Tubal surgery, when indicated, allows for natural conception and more than one pregnancy can be achieved as a result.

It should be considered the first-line treatment for proximal tubal disease, reversal of sterilization and fimbrial adhesions.

IVF should be offered to those with severe distal tubal disease and severe endometriosis.

It may also be indicated in patients who have not conceived within one year following microsurgery.

In patients with patent tubes following microsurgery, GIFT may be performed.

More clinical experience can solve the dilemma of whether it is beneficial to perform GIFT or to offer IVF primarily to the patient.

Between January 1987 and December 1990 at the Jones Institute for Reproductive Medicine, the most common indications for IVF were tubal factors (57%).

Much of the discussion about the management of tubal disease has centered on the cost of ART versus tubal surgery.

Most authors agree that the cost of IVF is less than, or the same as, that of tubal surgery.

ART is the preferred method for women suffering from multiple tubal obstructions, after bilateral salpingectomy, or with extensive and dense pelvic adhesions.

The three-month cumulative probabilities of pregnancy after multiple IVF cycles were:

−33% in women with tubal factor younger than 35 years,

−25% in women with tubal factor older than 35 years,

−30% for women with multiple factors younger than 35 years, and

−14% for women with multiple factors older than 35 years.

Male Infertility

Male infertility has become as common as tubal factors as an indication for IVF.

Initially, male subfertility was treated using GIFT when couples had not responded to any other method of treatment, including IUI, and patent tubes were present.

However, the results show that the pregnancy outcome after GIFT in couples with severe male infertility is significantly lower than that following GIFT with normal sperm.

With the establishment of ICSI for couples with male infertility, most causes of male infertility can now be treated.

The majority of infertile males have oligospermia and/or low sperm motility and are subfertile rather than sterile.

In men with azoospermia, sperm cells obtained from the epididymis or by testicular biopsy may prove satisfactory for the ICSI technique.

The exceptional results of subzontal injection of the oocyte (SUZI), and more particularly ICSI, now raise the prospect of pregnancy being possible even when there are low numbers of sperm in the ejaculate, and bring to treatment focus some azoospermic men and men without antegrade ejaculate.

The advance in clinical results from SUZI and ICSI over earlier zona drilling and zona binding techniques appears to be giving better implantation potential to the embryos.

Technical factors critical for achieving high rates of fertilization and pregnancy include the use of standardized ICSI pipettes, the immobilization of sperm before injection, and the aspiration of a minimal amount of ooplasm before reinjection with the sperm.

ICSI is superior to other micromanipulation methods for alleviating male infertility.

However, there has been some concern regarding the abnormal fetal karyotypes.

In 1993, a single spermatozoon was injected into the ooplasm of oocytes with a fertilization rate of 64.2%, and this was not influenced by sperm morphology or motility.

Total and clinical pregnancy rates of 49.6% and 39.2%, respectively, per ET were reported.

This new development raises skepticism regarding the applicability of conventional semen parameters.

If normal embryos can be produced by ICSI, doubts regarding such theories as a natural selection process and the correlation of sperm head morphology and quality of the DNA arise.

Unexplained Infertility

Unexplained infertility can be defined to include those couples with more than two years of infertility with no abnormalities on repeated investigation of the fallopian tubes, ovulation, luteal phase, cervical mucus, semen, semen-mucus interaction or intercourse.

However, it should be noted that there are many couples who have minor abnormalities but no adequate explanation for their inability to conceive.

The duration of the infertility and the age of the patient are particularly important.

It should also be noted that a large number of patients enter IVF programs as "idiopathic infertility" but that during subsequent investigations and treatment, the cause of the infertility may become apparent.

Therefore, IVF has resulted in the diagnosis and treatment of idiopathic infertility.

Many empirical modalities have been suggested for the treatment of couples with unexplained infertility.

These include IUI, steroid and antibiotic therapy, bromocriptine, ovulation induction, combined treatments and ART.

The ESHRE multicenter trial was designed to compare the effectiveness of superovulation alone with superovulation with either IUI, GIFT, IVF or intraperitoneal insemination.

The pregnancy rates obtained in the trial were in excess of rates reported for untreated couples, and the mean pregnancy rates for the four invasive methods were similar.

However, the application of ART increased the chance of pregnancy by nearly two times beyond that obtained by superovulation alone.

General indications of IVF in unexplained infertility include the following:

−No success after 1 year of treatment, or

−No success after 3 to 6 cycles of IUI (for male factor infertility), or

−No success after 6 cycles of ovulation induction and IUI (for unexplained infertility or a combination of male and female infertility factors), or

−Overstimulation with gonadotropin ovulation induction leading to concerns about multiple gestation.

Ovulatory Disorders

Disorders of ovulation resistant to treatment by ovulation induction with either clomiphene citrate (CC) or urinary gonadotropins may respond to IVF.

The most common disorder of ovulation which may prove resistant is the polycystic ovary syndrome (PCOS).

The presenting symptom of patients with PCOS is often infertility due to chronic oligo- or anovulation, and the restoration of ovulatory function assumes paramount importance.

CC is the first line of treatment for chronic anovulation that accompanies PCOS.

However, if it fails, then conventional gonadotropin therapy is indicated.

Unfortunately, this therapy is associated with an increased spontaneous abortion rate, multiple gestation rate and ovarian hyperstimulation syndrome (OHSS).

Although today's readily available monitoring technology (ultrasonography and rapid serum estrogen measurements) make gonadotropin therapy safer in terms of multiple gestation and OHSS, they are both time intensive and expensive and these complications lead to a high rate of cycle cancellation.

The use of IVF in patients with PCOS enables:

−Controlled ovarian hyperstimulation (COH) in conjunction with GnRH down regulation.

−Aspiration of all ovarian follicles present.

−The option of freeze/thawing all resultant embryos and subsequent transfer in a non-stimulation cycle.

−The resultant decrease in the incidence of OHSS.

IVF is being increasingly used in association with ovulatory disorders and in particular PCOS.

However, despite the high pregnancy rate from transfer of embryos, there is a high first trimester abortion rate as well.

Endometriosis

The etiology of infertility in endometriosis is unclear, and a multitude of factors are involved.

In advanced (stage III and IV) endometriosis, pelvic adhesions distort pelvic anatomy and interfere with the reproductive process.

In mild (stage I and II) endometriosis, the mechanism of infertility is less clear.

These effects are relative and individually variable, and some women with endometriosis have no infertility problems.

A variety of mechanisms through which limited endometriosis may lower fertility has been postulated:

−Ovulatory dysfunction, the prevalence of which would seem to be similar in endometriosis and in the infertile population in general.

−Alterations in gamete/ET.

−Anti-fertility effects of the peritoneal fluid, which may affect sperm motility/survival, fertilization, gamete interaction and early embryo development.

−Peritoneal macrophages causing increased sperm phagocytosis, decreased motility and impaired ability to penetrate the egg.

−An anti-implantation effect related to evidence for antigen-antibody reaction in the uterine cavity of women with endometriosis which may be the mechanism of infertility and recurrent miscarriages.

Most of the mechanisms implicated in endometriosis should be corrected by IVF.

Aspiration of the eggs with ultrasound-guided needles, IVF, early embryonic development in the laboratory and ET should correct problems caused by ovulatory dysfunction, abnormal fertilization, failure of early embryonic development.

One would, therefore, expect IVF pregnancy rates to be comparable in patients with and without endometriosis.

There is no agreement in the literature regarding the benefits of medical pretreatment of endometriosis before the IVF cycles; the most common medical pretreatments were either danazol or GnRH.

Immunological Infertility

Immunological factors may operate at almost every step in the human reproductive process.

Some of the cases of immune infertility could result from destruction of gametes by antisperm antibodies or by preventing embryo cleavage and early development.

The mechanism by which the presence of antisperm antibodies interferes with human reproduction has never been documented clearly and there is no absolute proof that immunity to sperm can cause subfertility.

Theoretically, ART should bypass the early stages of fertilization, during which sperm are exposed to the antisperm antibodies within the female genital tract, and alleviate subfertility related to female immunological infertility.

Female patients with significant levels of antisperm antibodies in the serum had similar fertilization rates after IVF when compared with patients with no significant levels and suggest that females' antisperm antibodies may not hinder fertilization in-vitro.

In this particular group of conditions, ART has not yet caused a dramatic change and the benefits derived from it remain unclear.

Preimplantation Genetic Diagnosis (PGD)

PGD is indicated when there is the potential for transmission of an undesired genetic defect.

TECHNIQUE OF IVF

PRE-CYCLE ASSESSMENT

Prior to IVF, a semen analysis and assessment of the fallopian tubes and normalcy of the uterine cavity should be performed.

Semen Analysis

Sperm concentration, motility and morphology should be optimized and pyospermia treated, if present.

Pyospermia (white blood cells in the semen) suggests infection, and a course of antibiotics should be given prior to sperm use with IVF.

A visit to a male infertility specialist prior to the treatment cycle may be indicated for men with a suboptimal semen analysis.

Assessment of Fallopian Tubes

Pre-cycle assessment of the fallopian tubes is usually done with a hysterosalpingogram (HSG).

If there is evidence of hydrosalpinges (fluid in the fallopian tubes), data indicate they should be removed or proximally blocked before IVF treatment if this can be done safely.

The presence of a hydrosalpinx with communication to the uterine cavity decreases the pregnancy rate by 50%.

Although the exact reason for this is not clear, it is hypothesized that the fluid causes mechanical flushing and loss of the embryos or contains inflammatory mediators that negatively impact implantation.

The success rate with GIFT in women with tubal disease is not greater than with IVF, and the risk of tubal pregnancy is higher; therefore, IVF is most appropriate with significant tubal abnormalities.

The success rate increases to normal after tubal repair or salpingectomy; occlusion of the proximal tube seems to be equally efficacious.

Endometrial integrin is reduced in many patients with hydrosalpinx and revers to a normal pattern after salpingectomy.

Spontaneous pregnancy can occur when a unilateral hydrosalpinx is removed or repaired.

It has been suggested that only hydrosalpinges which are visible on transvaginal ultrasound should be removed.

However, hydrosalpinges enlarge during stimulation and may become visible only during the IVF cycle.

Assessment of Uterine Cavity

Specialized assessments of the uterine cavity are required depending on the clinical situation.

For a cycle using cryopreserved embryos, uterine assessment should show an endometrial lining thickness of $\geq$6-8 mm on ultrasound at time of frozen-thawed ET.

While more controversial in fresh IVF treatment cycles, endometrial lining thickness (and, potentially, lining appearance) appears to predict pregnancy and live birth rates.

In general, a thicker endometrium with a trilaminar pattern is preferred:

−The endometrial lumen is demonstrated by the central echogenic line,

−The hypoechogenic layer representing the edematous endometrial functionalis, and

−An outer echogenic area representing the endometrium basalis.

There are very few successful pregnancies when endometrial lining thickness is <6 mm at the time of progesterone supplementation and frozen-thawed ET.

In addition, ovaries should have no active corpus luteum and the progesterone level must be <3 ng/mL.

Endogenous progesterone production will alter the window of implantation for a frozen-thawed embryo, and such cycles must be delayed or cancelled.

For fresh embryo cycles, prior to starting gonadotropin stimulation, ovaries should have no productive ovarian follicles; that is, no baseline follicles measuring 15 mm or larger; the estradiol level must be less than 50 to 80 pg/mL.

Large, dominant ovarian follicles will prevent stimulation of other ovarian follicles by the gonadotropin medications during a fresh IVF cycle; thus the cycle must be delayed or cancelled if these are present.

A pre-cycle trial or mock ET or uterine "sounding" should be done to predict and avoid difficult ET.

If a cervix is difficult to traverse at the time of the mock ET, there are a number of strategies that can be used prior to the cycle start.

These include use of transabdominal ultrasound guidance at the time of ET, placement of laminaria to dilate the cervix prior to cycle start, cervical dilation using sequential dilators prior to cycle start, or use of a stylet (a stiff wire guide within an outer flexible catheter) at the time of ET.

Transvaginal ultrasound with or without saline infusion can identify intracavitary polyps or fibroids, which should be removed prior to start.

The presence of these lesions is associated with a lower success rate in IVF cycles.

Significant polyps or myomata are often easily visualized; a sonohysterogram or hysteroscopy should be done if there is a further question of uterine disease.

A randomized, controlled study has shown a higher pregnancy rate following hysteroscopic excision of small (16 mm) polyps, underlining the importance of a thorough evaluation of the uterine cavity.

Other studies have suggested that the polyp excision itself may enhance implantation from the healing process.

A randomized study showed that a biopsy done in the cycle immediately preceding IVF was associated with increased implantation.

Submucous fibroids markedly reduce the pregnancy rate with IVF; studies have been conflicting regarding the role of intramural myomas, with some studies showing a significant reduction of outcome and other not showing an effect.

It is likely that intramural myomas reduce implantation, but the effect is probably small unless the uterine cavity is distorted.

Very large numbers would be required to accurately quantify such an effect; excision is advised if they are large or distort the cavity.

Generally, a uterine septum should be incised before going on to IVF because of the higher risk of spontaneous abortion.

Endometriosis

Even in the presence of mild endometriosis, quantitative defects of the secretory response of endometrial glandular cells and other endometrial abnormalities have been described.

Any endometriomal fluid should be kept separate from aspirates containing oocytes, and aspirating needles and pipettes should be changed.

Two randomized studies have shown that a 3-6 month course of GnRH agonist leading directly into IVF is associated with an increased pregnancy rate in women with stage III and IV endometriosis.

Hepatitis and HIV

Most programs screen for hepatitis and HIV for safety of personnel.

It would also be tragic to expend the amount of effort required to achieve an IVF pregnancy only to have the offspring at risk for a potentially fatal disease.

With hepatitis B, the female partner should be immunized; with HIV, sperm separation and ICSI is being used by some programs to avoid transmission of the virus.

Sexual Dysfunction

Rarely, anxiety can lead to total inability to provide a semen specimen on the day of retrieval.

Frozen husband's sperm has been found to yield a fairly normal rate of fertilization provided an increased number of sperm is added.

Personal Habits

Smoking increases the rate of spontaneous abortion. It is recommended that all women stop smoking before having IVF.

A study of caffeine use found that intake of 2 mg (equivalent to one cup of decaf coffee) or less was associated with the highest pregnancy rate with IVF.

Although not confirmed by other studies, avoiding caffeine is a simple measure to undertake.

Studies on alcohol and fertility are conflicting, with some showing impaired fertility with small amounts of alcohol; whereas in one study, wine drinkers had a shorter time to conception.

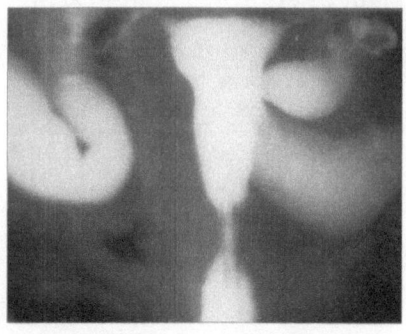

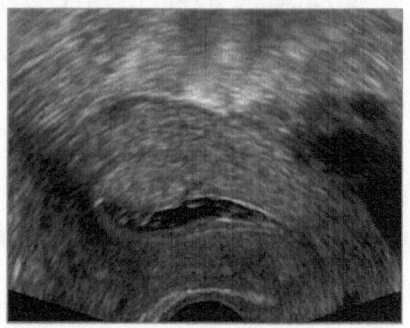

Bilateral Hydrosalpinx   **Endometrial Polyp**

Pre-cycle Assessment

CONTROLLED OVARIAN HYPERSTIMULATION

COH is frequently used with IVF cycles, as it does improve pregnancy rates.

Exact protocols vary by clinic, but involve the use of injectable gonadotropins.

The use of an oral contraceptive prior to treatment may minimize cycle cancellation and allow for greater control of cycle management.

A commonly-used stimulation protocol uses a combination of GnRH agonists and gonadotropins.

Natural cycle IVF (using no medications) and minimal stimulation protocols (using oral ovulation-induction agents) are other possibilities, but the yield of oocytes and embryos, and thus pregnancy rates, are significantly lower.

These alternatives are useful for avoiding OHSS and decreasing the chances of a multiple pregnancy.

The aim of all stimulation protocols is to induce the development of a cohort of equidominant follicles in both ovaries.

The success rate in any one IVF cycle has been clearly shown to be increased form 4.2% in a natural cycle to 17% in a stimulated cycle where more than one embryo is transferred.

An increased number of eggs at the time of oocyte retrieval is directly linked to a significant improvement in pregnancy rates.

Stimulation regimens are designed with the following aims:

−To prevent premature luteinization.

−To prevent spontaneous ovulation.

−To improve endometrial response.

−To allow greater flexibility for ambulatory patient management, with reduced cycle monitoring, and the giving of injections at home.

Modifications to stimulation protocols are continually being reviewed:

−The protocol needs to be tailored to each individual patient in order to maximize the prospect of success whilst minimizing possible complications.

−Emphasis is given to a team approach in the making of decisions regarding stimulation; usually the patient's clinician, liaising with the nurse practitioner directly involved with the patient's care, and the embryologist, if necessary in consultation with a specialist endocrinologist, will meet to decide the most appropriate protocol.

−Varied protocols of COH have been developed within different centers based on the use of the agents described; ongoing modifications will occur depending on the patient's response, newer agents and the results of treatment.

COH Regimens for IVF

IVF therapy has become increasingly simplified in recent years.

The use of GnRH agonists and antagonists with gonadotropins has resulted in greater ease of planning the supervoulation stimulation than was possible with the earlier use of CC with gonadotropin, that regimen had to be monitored carefully in order to predict and prevent the occurrence of an endogenous prevoulatory LH surge.

In the absence of GnRH controlled cycles there is a cancellation rate of 15% because oocyte retrieval has to be performed 26 hours after the detection of the endogenous surge and this often meant that oocyte collections were performed at night and at weekends.

When GnRH agonists or antagonists are used, the oocyte retrieval can be precisely timed to occur 34 hours after the administration of hCG.

hCG acts as a surrogate for the normal mid-cycle LH surge, and causes resumption of meiosis within the oocytes and their preparation for fertilization.

Furthermore, there is good evidence that the oocytes do not become overmature within follicles that are considered to be ready for collection and so the administration of hCG can be delayed to avoid oocyte collection at weekends.

Success rates appear to be better when GnRH agonists are used and the rates of miscarriage, especially in patients with PCOS, appear to be reduced.

Most stimulation regimens commence the day after menses has started (i.e., day 2) for practical reasons.

A day 1 start is acceptable but often not practical as most clinics like to communicate with their patients when they are about to start treatment.

Alternatively, the combined oral contraceptive pill can be used to program the cycle.

Pituitary desensitization "downregulatin" has occurred when the serum concentration of LH is <5 IU/L and that of estradiol <50 pg/mL (progesterone, if measured, should be <3 mmol/L).

hCG or recombinant LH is given to trigger oocyte maturation when the largest follicle reaches at least 18 mm in diameter and there are at least two others >17 mm; oocyte collection is performed 35 hours later; ET occurs approximately 48 hours after oocyte collection.

Luteal support commences the day of ET and is usually given as progesterone suppositories or i.m. injections and continued until the day of the pregnancy test.

Some continue luteal support up to 12 weeks' gestation, although this is unnecessary if progesterone pessaries have been used.

A disadvantage of the use of GnRH agonists is the 2 weeks or more lead-in to the therapy during which pituitary desensitization "down-regulation" is achieved before stimulation with gonadotropins can be commenced.

Pituitary desensitization is assessed by a combination of endometrial shedding and low serum concentrations of estradiol and LH (although ultrasound confirmation of a thin endometrium and quiescent ovaries is adequate without recourse to biochemistry).

Some clinics prefer to commence agonist therapy on day 21 of the cycle and suggest that desensitization occurs more rapidly than if it is commenced during menstruation – usually day 2.

A day 21 start, however, carries the risk of "rescuing" a corpus luteum with resultant functional cyst formation; a day 2 start virtually guarantees that the patient is not pregnant.

Combined oral contraceptive pill can be administered for between 2 and 3 weeks commencing on day 1 of the menstrual cycle.

This regimen allows scheduling of cycles in a busy clinic and also the use of the contraceptive pill minimizes the occurrence of ovarian cysts resulting from the GnRH agonist "flare".

The disadvantage, of course, is further prolongation of the treatment cycle.

The GnRH agonists can be administered intranasally, subcutaneously, or intramuscularly.

The shorter acting preparations can be used to induce a flare response, being commenced on day 1 of the cycle, with gonadotropin stimulation starting the following day.

The agonist is then either continued through to the day of hCG "short protocol" or given for 3 days only "ultrashort protocol".

The flare response can be utilized in those patients who have had a poor response in the past in order to try to maximize the response to stimulation – this it does to varying degrees.

It is, in fact, difficult to predict an individual's response to stimulation: young women and those with PCOS tend to respond well, while older patients and those with elevated baseline serum concentrations of FSH (>10 IU/L on most assays) respond less well.

CC and GnRH stimulation tests have been employed to improve the predictability of response but do not tend to be highly sensitive. An assessment of ovarian volume, antral follicle count and anti-Müllerian hormone (AMH) concentration have become popular in assessing ovarian reserve.

As with many aspects of current clinical practice, the evidence on which our therapy is based relies upon data from small trials.

Furthermore, different preparations, criteria for treatment, and protocols have been used, making comparison of studies difficult.

This has led to the use of meta-analyses of studies in order to provide firmer conclusions.

An early meta-analysis indicated that cycle cancellation rates had decreased and clinical pregnancy rates increased since the introduction of the "long" protocol of pituitary desensitization.

Ten studies were included in this analysis, with 914 agonist/gonadotropin cycles compared against 722 with CC and gonadotropins.

The clinical pregnancy rates per cycle started were significantly greater with agonist treatment and more oocytes collected.

With agonist use there was also a greater gonadotropin requirement by approximately 12 ampoules per cycle and a trend towards a higher rate of OHSS.

A more recent analysis of the different types of agonist regimen was been published in the Cochrane Database in which 26 trials met the inclusion criteria.

Those regimens that achieved pituitary desensitization produced the highest pregnancy rates and the luteal phase commencement of GnRH agonist was probably more advantageous than starting treatment in the follicular phase.

The advent of the third-generation GnRH antagonist enables us to dispense with pituitary densitization and commence ovarian stimulation on day 2, with the daily administration of an antagonist on day 6 of stimulation or once the leading follicle(s) has reached a diameter of 14 mm (usually day 6 or 7).

However, it appears that success rates are better when commenced on day 6 rather than using a flexible protocol.

GnRH antagonists act immediately to inhibit pituitary secretion of FSH and LH without the flare effect of antagonists or the need for 10 days' desensitization; an endogenous LH surge can be prevented, thereby allowing oocyte retrieval at the desired time.

GnRH antagonist cycles are certainly much shorter and more convenient for patients than the "long protocol" and many clinics are now increasingly using them.

Oocyte maturation prior to collection may be initiated with a single shot of a GnRH agonist rather than hCG – a strategy that was proposed to reduce the risk of OHSS because of the shorter half-life of the agonist compared with hCG; however pregnancy rates are lower and so the conventional use of hCG is recommended.

The use of GnRH antagonists may also reduce the total requirement for gonadotropins and obviate any need for luteal support.

GnRH antagonist cycles may be preferred because of their short duration and minimal side effects (for example, avoidance of symptoms of estrogen deficiency during pituitary desensitization).

There is no evidence that the type or dose of gonadotropin needs to be modified when using antagonists compared with agonist regimens.

Initial studies found pregnancy rates were approximately 5% lower than with GnRH agonist cycles, although it has been suggested that there is a "learning curve" in appreciating the optimal time to plan oocyte retrieval.

This is still an area of ongoing research encouraged by a recent meta-analysis, which concludes that there is a similar probability of a live birth when either GnRH agonists or antagonists are used.

1. Clomiphene citrate plus gonadotropins (hMG or FSH)

oocyte collection □

menses (day 1)

clomiphene 100 mg per day
day 2 for 5 days

gonadotropin stimulation from day 4 to day of hCG

hCG □

2. Long GnRH agonist protocols

a. Luteal phase start (i.e., 7 days after presumed day of ovulation)

oocyte collection □

ovulation   menses

GnRH agonist day 21

drop dose, continue to
day of hCG

gonadotropins to day of hCG

hCG □

b. Follicular phase start

oocyte collection □

menses

GnRH agonist starts day 2 until
"downregulation,"
usually 14 days

drop dose, continue to
day of hCG

gonadotropins to day of hCG

hCG □

3. Short GnRH agonist protocal

oocyte collection □

menses (day 1)

GnRH agonist starts day 2 to day of hCG

gonadotropin stimulation from day 3 to day of hCG

hCG □

4. Ultra-short GnRH agonist protocol

oocyte collection □

menses (day 1)

GnRH agonist from
day 2 for 3 days

gonadotropin stimulation from day 3 to day of hCG

hCG □

5. GnRH antagonist protocol (a GnRH agonist can be given instead of hCG)

oocyte collection □

menses (day 1)

gonadotropin stimulation from day 2 to day of hCG

daily injection of antagonist when leading follicle 14 mm □

hCG □

COH Regimens

Gonadotropin Therapy for IVF

Gonadotropin therapy for the stimulation of superovulation can be with either human menopausal gonadotropin (hMG), which contains urinary-derived FSH and LH in differing proportions depending on the preparation, or with urinary-derived FSH alone, which is available for administration subcutaneously because of its higher purity.

The original sources of gonadotropins for therapeutic use were post-mortem pituitary extracts and the urine of postmenopausal women.

The former source was withdrawn because of cases of Creutzfeldt-Jakob disease, which occurred predominantly in Australia but was also reported in Europe.

The extraction and purification of postmenopausal urine were pioneered in Italy in the late 1940s to result in the production of hMG.

Twenty to thirty liters of postmenopausal urine were required to provide sufficient gonaodtropin for one cycle of hMG.

Through the 1960s the extraction process to remove non-specific co-purified proteins became more sophisticated, such that activity was increased 10 fold over the early preparations.

Greater purity produced fewer hypersensitivity reactions and less discomfort from the smaller volume of the injection.

Clinical trials comparing uFSH (urofollitropin) and highly purified FSH demonstrated equivalent ovulation and pregnancy rates.

Reduced hypersensitivity was reported, such that the subcutaneous route could be adopted for administration.

However, the problems of supply, collection, transport, storage, and processing of an ever increasing requirement of urine remained and the pharmaceutical companies have now utilized the technology of genetic engineering to produce biosynthetic preparations.

This process has resulted in an unlimited supply of highly stable therapeutic preparations with a high specific activity.

The advent of the recombinantly derived gonadotropins has broadened the scope of therapeutic agents and resulted in a potentially unlimited supply.

To date there are two recombinant FSH preparations: follitropin alfa (Gonal-F, Serono) and follitropin beta (Puregon, Organon).

In discussing the benefits of a gonadotropin preparation one has to consider clinical efficacy, side effects and cost-effectiveness.

Clinical efficacy includes the ability to stimulate folliculogenesis, the production of mature oocytes, appropriate steroidogenesis for endometrial development and, in the context of IVF, sufficient quality pre-embryos and, ultimately, good rates of pregnancy.

Monitoring the Treatment Cycle

The monitoring of follicular response to superovulation requires a combination of parameters.

Specifically, there needs to be vaginal ultrasound assessment of follicular size and number, and measurements of plasma estradiol, LH and progesterone levels need to be ascertained

The patient's history and current treatment are scrutinized together with the current results.

Decisions concerning changes in management, cycle cancellation alteration in drug dosage, timing of hCG and oocyte recovery are conveyed promptly to the patient.

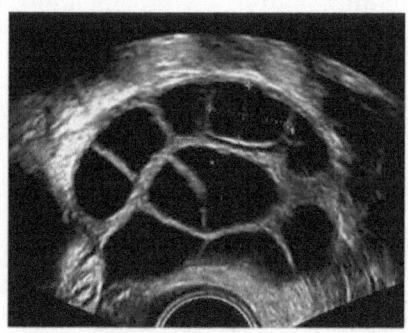

COH Ultrasound

Criteria for Cancellation:

−Abnormal findings seen on ultrasound scan.

−Falling estradiol levels despite increased stimulation.

−Estradiol greater than 6000 pg/mL; if this hyperstimulation occurs, consider continuing GnRH agonist down regulation until the ovaries are quiescent.

Ovarian Reserve

Ovarian reserve, or the number of release oocytes, declines with ovarian age, which does not always equate with the age of the woman.

As ovarian reserve declines, so too does the chromosomal integrity of the ovulated oocytes, so that there is a rise in the rates of miscarriage and fetal chromosomal abnormalities.

There are number of tests of ovarian reserve but all have limitations.

Measurement of ovarian hormones (e.g. estradiol inhibin, anti-Mullerian hormone) to some degree reflects ovarian age.

The response of the ovary to COH by gonadotropins is the essential test of ovarian function but provides only a retrospective analysis rather than a prospective indication of the likely response to treatment that can be used to determine the starting dose or stimulation regimen.

A baseline measurement of serum FSH concentration, usually on day 3 of the cycle, is a fairly good predictor of ovarian reserve.

As the ovary fails, the FSH begins to rise in the follicular phase of the cycle.

When the FSH is elevated there is a greater likelihood of monthly fluctuations in FSH concentration than when the FSH is normal.

A fluctuating baseline FSH level is indicative of already compromised ovarian function.

There is little to be gained by waiting to start treatment in a cycle in which the FSH level is closer to the normal range.

An ultrasound scan of the ovaries may also be helpful; ovarian response has been positively correlated with ovarian volume and the number of antral follicles.

The appearance of polycystic ovaries, whether or not there is overt PCOS, indicates that the ovaries are likely to respond sensitively to stimulation, with the likely production of many follicles, although not necessarily with an equivalent number of oocytes of good quality.

Stimulation tests have been evaluated with the aim of enhancing the predictability of ovarian response to superovulation.

CC (100 mg) can be administered from day 5 and the serum FSH concentration measured on days 3 and 10.

It is thought that in response to CC the day 10 FSH rises before there is a rise in the basal day 3 FSH concentrations.

Ovarian reserve can also be assessed by stimulation with a GnRH agonist.

In practice a baseline serum FSH concentration on day 3 of the cycle usually suffices and if it is elevated it should be repeated on at least one occasion.

It is recommended that a baseline endocrine profile (FSH, LH, thyroid function) be repeated annually in women attending the fertility clinic, or more frequently if there is a change in the patient's menstrual cycle or an expectedly poor response to ovarian stimulation.

The recommended starting dose for stimulation in superovulation regimens for IVF is 150-225 units of FSH or hMG in women with a normal serum FSH concentration under the age of 38 years.

Women over the age of 38 years may be given higher doses depending upon their baseline serum FSH concentration and antral follicle count.

In women with an elevated baseline FSH or those who have responded poorly in a previous cycle (i.e., fewer than 5 oocytes collected) the dose is increased to a maximum of 450 units.

There appears to be no benefit in using higher doses, neither does there appear to be significant benefit in increasing the dose of stimulation mid-treatment after follicles have been recruited.

If a baseline ultrasound scan indicates the presence of polycystic ovaries (whether or not there are signs of the PCOS) we reduce the starting dose to 150 units, depending upon age and previous response to stimulation.

If an exuberant response to stimulation is anticipated ultrasound monitoring is started earlier (day 6 or 7 of stimulation) and may reduce the dose of FSH as soon as follicles > 10 mm have been recruited.

The patient's response is reviewed after each cycle of treatment and the dose of stimulation adjusted according to the response obtained.

It is prefer to use the lowest dose that achieves the desired response to reduce the risk of ovarian hyperstimulation.

OOCYTE RETRIEVAL

Oocyte retrieval requires sensitive timing. When lead follicles, the largest, are 18-22 mm in diameter, hCG is given to trigger oocyte maturation.

A GnRH agonist may be an alternative to trigger oocyte maturation in order to minimize the risk of OHSS.

However, this should be used only in cycles in which GnRH was not used for stimulation.

Oocyte retrieval is scheduled for 34-36 hours after hCG. This may be delayed safely for up to 38 hours if a GnRH agonist is used.

Ovulation may occur if oocyte retrieval is delayed too long after hCG administration.

Usually, one dose of prophylactic antibiotics is given before, during or after the procedure.

Some programs delay antibiotics until post-procedure due to concerns about potential negative effects on oocytes.

Intravenous sedation ranges from light to deep, depending on patient needs.

Hospital-based IVF programs are better able to perform deep sedation, regional anesthesia (in the case of contraindications to deep sedation), and/or general anesthesia if needed.

The vagina and perineum are cleansed with sterile saline with or without antibiotics.

Povidone-iodine and other antiseptics are detrimental to the oocyte and should not be used.

Ultrasound-guided transvaginal aspiration is the most common method, and all accessible follicles are drained.

Alternative means of accessing ovaries are sometimes necessary due to anatomic barriers; on occasion, the uterine wall must be traversed. Rarely, transvesical or transabdominal approaches are necessary.

Over the past years, the technique for oocyte retrieval has evolved from being a laparoscopic procedure, lasting an hour or more, to a procedure involving ultrasound-guided needle aspiration and taking approximately 20 minutes.

The laparoscopic approach involved a full relaxant general anesthesia; follicles were punctured and fluid aspirated using a stainless steel needle of 23 cm length with an internal diameter of 2.0 mm and an external diameter of 2.2 mm.

The problems encountered in this technique, apart from the morbidity associated with laparoscopy, included the obese patient where entry into the abdomen was difficult, adhesions making visualization unclear, bleeding within and from the follicle due to direct trauma, and follicular leakage.

The first use of ultrasound-guided percutaneous follicle aspiration was reported in 1982, with an oocyte recovery rate of 50% per patient.

The needle used had an internal diameter of 0.6 mm and was therefore less traumatic.

The next advancement and refinement came with the switch to ultrasound-guided needle aspiration per vaginal.

Quite apart from the benefits to a patient of this less invasive procedure, the number of eggs retrieved at oocyte collection increases.

This was because ultrasound affords greater accuracy in needle-tip localization, and also follicles within the ovary which would normally have been missed by the blind searching of the laparoscopic needle could be clearly seen by ultrasound, and directly aspirated.

Vaginal ultrasound needle follicle aspiration affords a dual benefit to the patient when compared to laparoscopy in terms of a reduced morbidity and ease of aspiration of previously unrecognized follicles within the ovary.

It is important that the ultrasound image clearly shows the major structures to be avoided at the time of needle aspiration.

In particular, the relationship of the ovary to blood vessels, uterus and loops of bowel must be noted to enable a trajectory for the needle to be selected so that its path through the pelvis is atraumatic.

A 17-gauge disposable single-channel aspiration needle, 31 cm in length, is used.

The bevel of the needle is set at 45 degrees with an ultrasound-identifiable mark on the tip to aid visualization.

Before use it is inspected to ensure that it is sharp, thus minimizing the risk of tearing of a follicle when introduced.

Teflon tubing, continuous from the needle bevel to a silicone bung, delivers the aspirate into 10 mL tissue culture tubes.

A simple system of heating blocks placed in a specially adapted test tube holder with space for a Pyrex container of flushing medium and a glass syringe has been devised to allow the temperature of the system to remain constant at 37 degrees Celsius.

A sufficient length of Teflon tubing also runs from the silicone bung to the aspiration pump connection.

The pump is a foot-pedal-operated Kmar-2000 vacuum regulator to allow the vacuum pressure to be selected accurately; for routine follicle aspiration, a pressure of minus 17 kPa is chosen.

The aspirating system is checked to be operational by sucking a small amount of culture medium through the needle into a culture tube.

Follicles are aspirated in a sequential fashion from largest to smallest as this will reveal the previously hidden smaller follicles within the ovary.

In most cases it is not necessary to withdraw the needle from the ovary, but rather to change its position within the ovary to go from one follicle to the next.

If the needle may block due to blood and debris, it should be withdrawn and reverse flush down the needle into a culture tube is usually all that is required to clear it.

Culture tubes are examined immediately by an embryologist and oocytes can be quickly identified.

The surgeon is able to watch the progress of the collection by means of a camera connected to the embryologist microscope and relayed to a monitor in the operating theatre.

Individual follicle flushing has been largely superseded by the vaginal technique where all follicles are visualized and drained.

In cases where folliculogenesis has been suboptimal and only a few follicles are present, follicle flushing may be required.

An appropriately sterilized glass syringe with needle tip, filled with flushing medium (Herpes buffered culture solution), is inserted into the flared end of the Teflon tubing coming from the aspiration needle.

The approximate follicular volume is inserted and then aspirated, and this procedure may be repeated up to six times to retrieve the oocyte.

The rate of risks and complications for oocyte retrieval is very small, less than 1%.

These include: infection, damage to bowel, bladder, vasculature, failure to retrieve any oocytes, inability to access the ovary or ovaries, intra-ovarian or intra-peritoneal bleeding, and the risks of anesthesia.

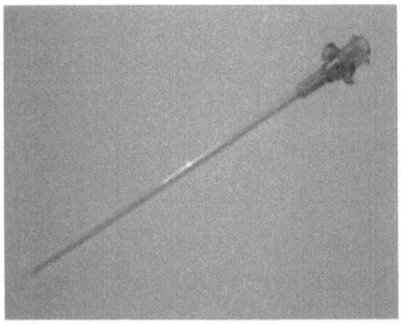

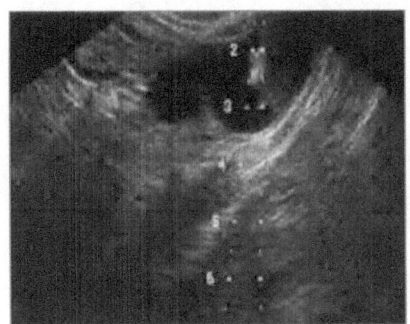

OPU Needle   **OPU Ultrasound**

Oocyte Retrieval

OOCYTE MATURATION

Oocyte maturation assessment in the laboratory is done by removal or spreading of the cumulus, that is, the surrounding granulosa cells, to directly visualize the oocyte.

The stage of maturation is based on the presence of a polar body and germinal vesicle.

Assessment based on cumulus cells is often inaccurate and could lead to premature insemination and failed fertilization.

Prophase I (PI) / Germinal Vesicle (GV)

The most immature oocytes are in Prophase I or Germinal Vesicle stage and have a germinal vesicle (nucleus) present but no polar body.

– Up to 30% of oocytes may be immature at the time of retrieval.

– The oocytes have 4N DNA in the nucleus, that is, 2N chromosomes, each with 2 chromatids.

– They may progress to Metaphase II in culture, but will not fertilize while immature.

– These oocytes have the lowest pregnancy potential.

Metaphase I (MI)

Oocytes in Metaphase I have no polar body or germinal vesicle.

– This stage is intermediate maturation and there are 2N chromosomes, each with 2 chromatids, thus the 4N quantity of DNA in the oocyte.

−More time in culture is needed for maturation, though this does not always occur.

−Insemination is done after maturation as the fertilization rate and pregnancy potential is higher.

Metaphase II (MII)

Retrieved oocytes are fully mature, at Metaphase II (MII) of maturation; the first polar body is present, and there is no germinal vesicle.

−Fully mature oocytes have 1N number of chromosomes, each with 2 chromatids. Thus the oocyte has a 2N quantity of DNA. The same is true of the first polar body.

−At this stage, reduction division has not yet been completed.

−Insemination should be done within 3-5 hours for the best chance of fertilization and optimal pregnancy potential.

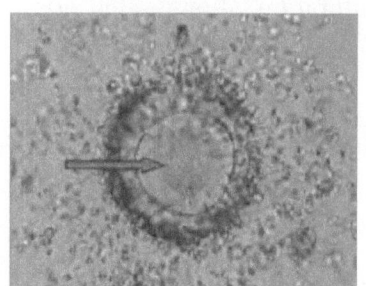
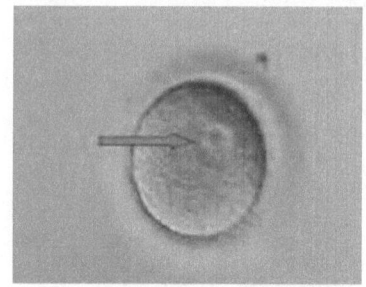

Prophase I (PI)

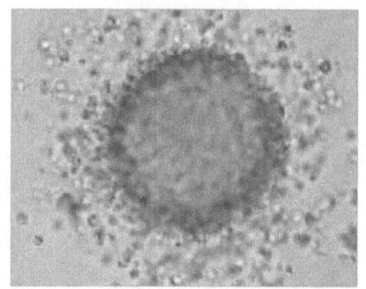
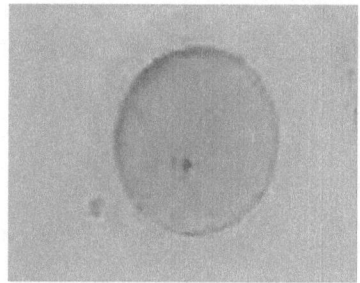

Metaphase I (MI)

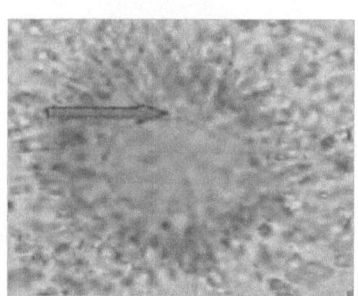
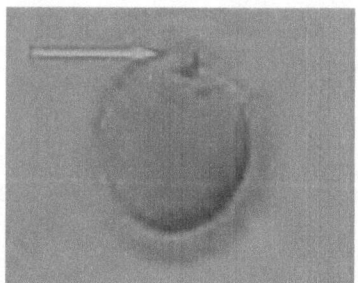

Metaphase II (MII)

Oocyte Maturation

SPERM PREPARATION

The objective of ART sperm preparation techniques is to obtain sperm with the highest potential for oocyte fertilization in a timely, cost-effective fashion.

The initial sample is typically collected into a sterile disposable plastic jar through masturbation, although alternative methods of collection are possible, as are surgical interventions.

Prior to preparation of sperm, the semen is allowed to liquefy through the actions of proteolytic enzymes originating from the prostate. Failure to liquefy within one hour is abnormal.

Preparation of the sample typically can take place within 15-30 minutes after collection.

Commonly employed methods of sperm preparation for ART include centrifugation, swim-up, density gradient centrifugation, and gel chromatography.

None of these methods is ideal for all ART indications; therefore, all of these methods are currently used in clinical ART practice.

Centrifugation

Simple wash, centrifugation and resuspension of sperm is the oldest method for preparing sperm.

The basic steps of this method include diluting the sperm with culture medium, centrifuging the sample, and resuspending the resulting pellet with the sperm for use.

The advantages of this method are that it is quick and inexpensive; however, there is concern that this method exposes sperm to damaging substances in the seminal fluid, including reactive oxygen species that could adversely affect the function of sperm in-vitro.

This method is commonly used for IUI. In addition, the technique does not remove insoluble material in the ejaculate.

Swim-Up

Similar to the centrifugation method of sperm preparation, the swim-up technique has been used for many years.

Several variations of this method have been described, but basically the seminal plasma is overlaid with culture medium and incubated for about 60 minutes.

During this time, active motile sperm swim from the seminal plasma into the culture medium, and the resulting sperm suspension then is centrifuged to concentrate the sperm.

This method is easy, cost-effective and usually results in the recovery of highly motile sperm.

However, this technique may not be suited for some cases, as many sperm may be lost in processing.

Another drawback of this method is that it takes approximately one hour to perform.

Despite these drawbacks, this method is the most commonly and successfully used for IVF and ICSI.

Density Gradient Centrifugation

The specimen is layered over a prepared discontinuous density gradient; colloidal silica density gradient (CSDG) is one commonly used density gradient.

The specimen and gradient are centrifuged, and bands of the density gradient, sperm and other material result.

The resulting layer at the bottom of the gradient contains the sperm, which is isolated and resuspended for use.

The main advantage of this technique is that it is quick; however, the drawbacks are that it may result in sperm with lower progressive motility and morphology compared with the swim-up method, although studies have yielded conflicting results.

Gel Chromatography

The specimen is layered over the top of columns containing gel particles, and while the specimen flows through the column, debris and dead sperm adhere to the gel and the resulting effluent is centrifuged and the pellet resuspended for use.

Similar to density-gradient method, gel chromatography method is quick.

Although reports vary, there is evidence that gel chromatography may yield sperm with higher motility than the density gradient method; however, the morphology of the sperm may be poorer.

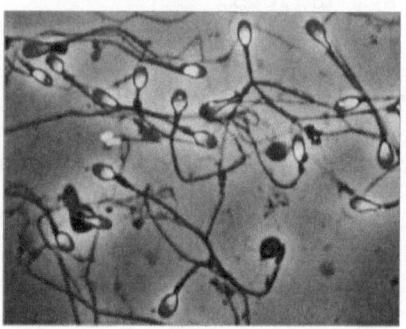

Normal Spermatozoa

INSEMINATION AND FERTILIZATION

A standard insemination of the retrieved oocytes is used when there is no significant male factor or concern for failed fertilization.

A fresh semen sample is collected by masturbation around time of retrieval and sperm are prepared to select highly motile sperm with normal morphology.

The prepared sperm are then incubated in protein-rich media to achieve capacitation, the process by which spermatozoa become capable of going through the acrosome reaction and fertilizing an oocyte.

Approximately 2 to 8 hours after retrieval, 50,000-100,000 motile sperm are incubated with each oocyte for 12 to 20 hours.

Fertilization occurs when hyaluronidase on the outer surface of the acrosome of the sperm facilitates migration through the cumulus-oocyte complex.

When a sperm encounters the zona pellucida, it undergoes the acrosome reaction, which breaks down the acrosomal membrane and releases a proteolytic enzyme that allows penetration.

The sperm head membrane binds to the sperm receptor, which is followed by fusion with the oocyte membrane.

Microvilli on the oocyte surface surround the sperm head and the oocyte releases cortical granules.

The zona pellucida then hardens and no other sperm can penetrate the oocyte membrane.

Release of cortical granules should prevent multiple sperm from entry, termed "polyspermy".

However, polyspermy does occur both naturally and in IVF and can lead to either failure of embryonic development or live birth with genetic abnormalities.

Abnormal fertilization is more likely to occur when oocytes (or sperm) are immature.

The fertilization process continues as the oocyte is "activated" and releases a second polar body.

The oocyte now has 1N quantity of DNA, that is, one set of 23 chromosomes, which is the full maternal contribution.

The male and female pronuclear form and approach each other; visualization of 2 pronuclei (and/or 2 polar bodies) in 6 to 20 hours suggests, but does not guarantee, normal fertilization.

A minority of zygotes will show 1 or more than 2 pronuclei, suggesting abnormal fertilization.

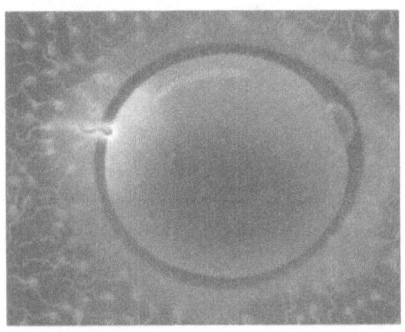 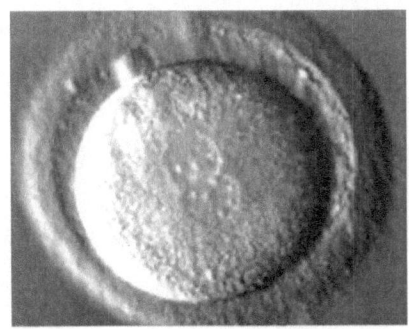

Fertilization Process   **Pronuclear Stage**

Insemination and Fertilization

EMBRYO DEVELOPMENT

Once the oocyte has fertilized, preembryos cleave in a series of mitotic divisions every 12-18 hours (or longer).

Each blastomere (individual cleavage cell) is "totipotent", that is, capable of developing an independent organism.

Preembryos usually progress in a series of even-numbered blastomere numbers, but asynchronous division is common and leads to odd-numbered blastomeres.

The goal of embryo culture is to replicate the conditions in the normal human fallopian tube, including temperature, electrolyte, protein, and carbohydrate concentrations; pH; osmolarity; and exposure to light.

Conditions are not standardized; some IVF labs have unique protocols and may make their own media, other labs use proprietary commercial media for which the precise components are viewed as "secret".

Some labs co-culture embryos with a patient's own endometrial cells; however the efficacy of this procedure is unproven.

For improvement of in-vitro embryo development, both media and culture conditions still need to be optimized.

Traditionally, preembryos have been transferred at the cleavage stage (2-3 days after fertilization).

Recent advances in culture media allow preembryo survival in culture to blastocyst stage.

In "sequential" culture media conditions, preembryos are transferred from media with non-essential amino acids and pyruvate to media with essential amino acids and glucose around day 3.

ET done at the blastocyst stage have higher implantation rates and potential for lower twin rates.

At the blastocyst stage, there is:

– Better ability to assess "true" viability after the embryonic genome has been activated,

– The ability to exclude embryos that have not progressed developmentally to this stage,

– The opportunity to simulate the natural day of embryonic arrival in the endometrial environment, and

– The time for preimplantation genetic testing.

Alternatively, some argue that embryos of lower quality may implant in the uterus if transferred on day 2-3 of culture but would not continue to develop in culture beyond that point.

This would represent a failed opportunity for this patient and these preembryos.

The process of cleavage changes to compaction at approximately the 8 to 16 cell stage.

Compaction involves change from individual cells to a solid mass of interconnected cells (which are no longer totipotent).

Morulae are compacted preembryos that develop between days 3-4 after insemination – they resemble mulberries.

About 24 hours after morula development, a central fluid-filled space develops, called the blastocele, and the preembryo is now called a blastocyst.

The inner cell mass of the blastocyst preembryo becomes the embryo, while the trophectoderm becomes the placenta.

Embryo Selection

Certain visible preembryo characteristics or morphologies have been associated with better pregnancy rates.

These characteristics or morphologies include:

– Appearance of polar bodies and cytoplasm in the prezygote stage;

– In the cleaving stages, the rate of cleavage, blastomere number and uniformity, cellular fragmentation, and presence or absence of multinucleation;

– The thickness of the zona pellucida at all stages; and

– The size of the blastocele and the appearance of the trophectoderm and inner cell mass in the blastocyst stage.

– Rates of chromosomal abnormality are also somewhat predicted by preembryo morphology.

Various scoring/grading systems have been based on these characteristics.

Scoring may be done daily or only on the day of transfer; scores may be used to dictate whether ET is performed on day 2 or 3 versus continuing in extended culture until the blastocyst stage.

While scores can help clinicians choose which preembryos to transfer to the uterus, they have not been proven to be predictive of live birth.

More studies are needed to determine the utility of scoring in embryo selection for transfer or cryopreservation and in predicting outcomes.

It is important to remember that only 25-35% of normal-appearing embryos actually implant and result in live births.

Comparative genomic hybridization to test for aneuploidy of embryos is an experimental, but promising, adjunct to morphologic assessment in selecting embryos with the best prognosis for live birth.

Cleavage Arrest

About 10 to 15% of preembryos permanently stop cleaving; this usually occurs at the 2-4 cell stage.

This may be due to self-arrest to prevent further development of chromosomally abnormal preembryos, self-arrest to prevent further development of preembryos with inadequate telomere length, or inadequate maternal genetic transcripts to handle the demands of development and the microenvironment.

Arrested development also occurs in natural conceptions; although estimates vary, about 30 to 60% of conceptions do not survive past week 12 of gestation.

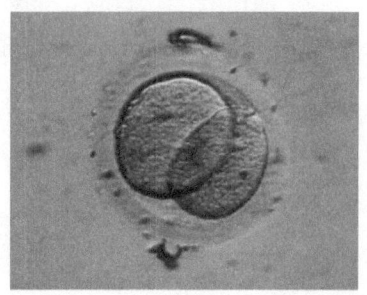

2-Cell Stage

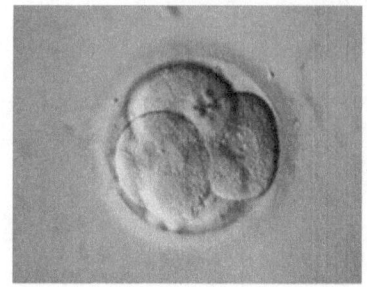

4-Cell Stage

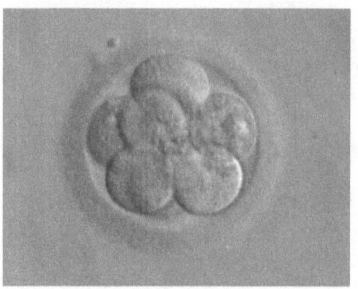

8-Cell Stage

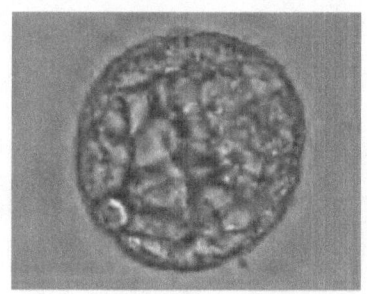

Morula

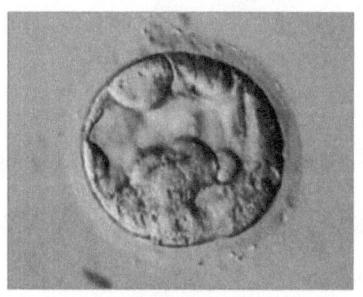

Blastocyst

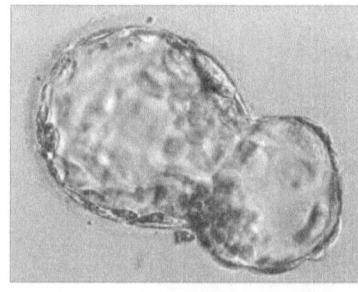

Hatching Blastocyst

Embryo Development

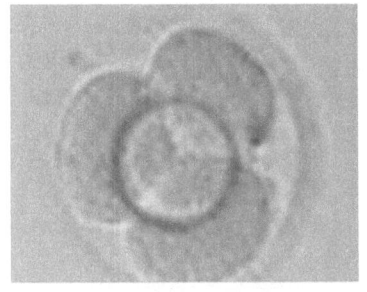

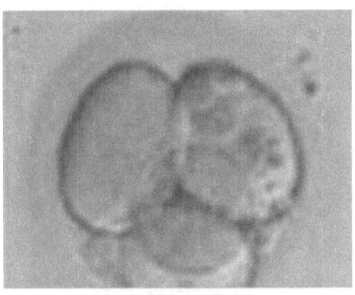

0% Fragmentation   **<10% Fragmentation**

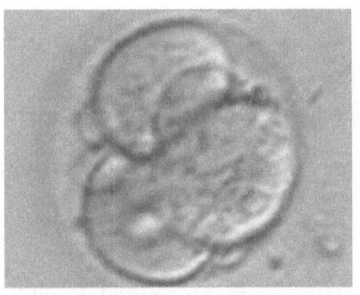

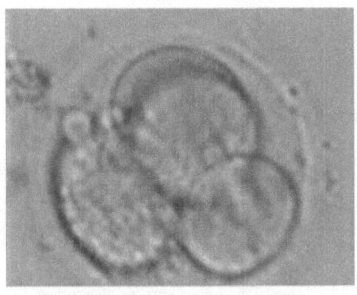

11-20% Fragmentation   **21-50% Fragmentation**

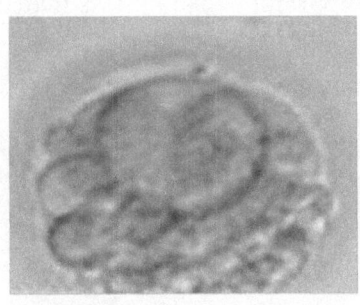

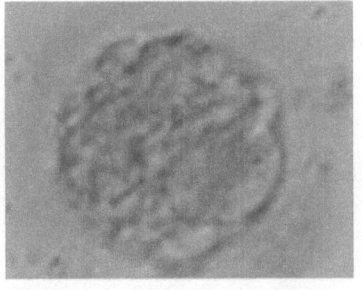

>50% Fragmentation   **100% Fragmentation**

Embryo Grading

EMBRYO TRANSFER

ET is most commonly performed 3 days after insemination at the cleaving stage.

The best pregnancy rates occur with preembryos containing 6-8 uniform blastomeres and little fragmentation.

Improved techniques using extended culture media have increased the use of blastocyst-stage transfers, which are performed 5 days after insemination.

This is most successful with preembryos containing an expanded blastocele, compact inner cell mass, uniform multicellular trophectoderm, and thin zona pellucida.

Recall that there are benefits and disadvantages to the use of blastocyst transfer.

The number of embryos to transfer is an important decision; less than 5% of the time, monozygotic twinning can occur.

This appears to have an association with extended culture to blastocyst stage.

Otherwise, an undesired outcome of multiple gestation is directly associated with number of embryos transferred.

The choice of number of embryos to transfer should be based on the patient's age, quality of preembryos, prior response to IVF treatment, and any medical co-morbidities or anatomical limitations.

In an effort to reduce the incidence of high-order multiple births, the ASRM has published guidelines to assist patients and ART programs in determining the appropriate number of embryos for transfer.

Prognosis is determined as favorable or unfavorable based on characteristics of the patient, such as number of IVF cycles, age, embryo quality and number of embryos available for cryopreservation.

For example, the recommendation for a <35-year-old woman with a favorable prognosis is for transfer of 1 blastocyst-stage embryo.

In contrast, a >35-year-old who has had unsuccessful IVF cycles could have up to 4 embryos transferred at cleavage stage, or up to 3 transferred at blastocyst stage.

Transcervical ET

Transcervical ET is by far the most commonly used procedure; the treatment cycle should be preceded by a trial or "mock" ET to anticipate any difficulty.

It may be helpful to wipe away excess cervical mucus prior to ET; a soft, flexible catheter is inserted through the cervix and the embryo(s) are gently expelled about 1-1.5 cm from the fundus.

Atraumatic ET with no uterine contractions and no resulting blood on the catheter tip are the most successful.

Success rates appear improved with the use of transabdominal ultrasound guidance at time of transfer.

Ultrasound guidance ensures optimal embryo location and may assist in problem-solving in the case of a difficult transfer.

Criteria for successful catheter design include the following:

−Ease of handling.

−Passage through an undilated cervix.

−Non embryo-toxic.

−Appropriate markings for depth of insertion within the uterus.

−Catheter tip detectable on ultrasound.

The catheter comprises an outer catheter, which acts as a sleeve to guide the cannula containing the embryos into the uterus, and is made of polyurethane with a polypropylene hub.

The inner embryo cannula is made of Teflon with a silicone hub, and measures 30 cm in length and 1 mm in diameter.

The outer catheter is introduced through the cervix to the internal os by means of a metal stilette, which affords rigidity and flexibility.

The patient is admitted to the operating room on the day surgery unit; the ET is performed without anesthesia; the patient is placed in a slight Trendelenberg position with her feet resting on elevated lithotomy poles, giving approximately 30 degrees of hip flexion.

The embryologist checks the identification of the patient and confirms the number of embryos to be transferred.

A bivalve speculum is inserted and the cervix exposed; mucus is cleansed from the cervix using peanut swabs soaked in culture medium; no antiseptic is used.

The outer sleeve of the catheter is introduced into the cervix and advanced to the internal os; the guide wire is removed and the sleeve advanced to the 5 cm mark.

After correct placement of the sleeve the embryologist is signaled to load the cannula.

A 0.02 mL of air is drawn into a 1 mL syringe and the cannula attached. A 3/il column of media is introduced into the cannula, 2/A of air is then introduced.

The embryos in culture medium (3/il) are drawn into the cannula followed by 2/A of air.

The tip of the cannula is sealed by dipping it into media and is pulled back into its sterile packaging and taken into the operating theatre.

The surgeon then introduces the cannula via the catheter sleeve into the uterus to the 5 cm mark.

The embryos are released into the uterus by gentle pressure on the plunger.

Transmyometrial ET

Although rarely used, a transmyometrial procedure using ultrasound guidance is an option if the cervix has been removed or is impassable.

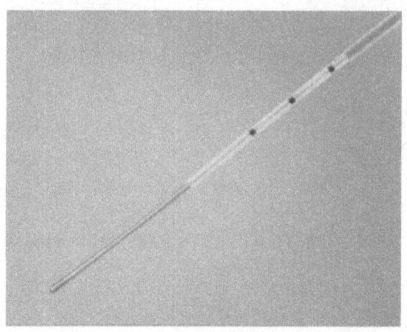 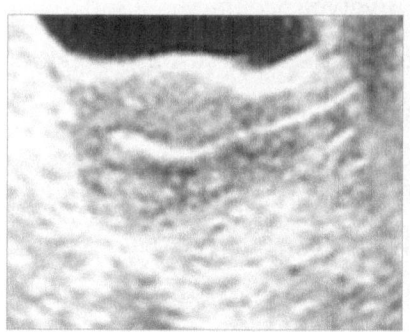

ET Catheter   **ET Ultrasound**

Embryo Transfer

POST-EMBRYO TRANSFER

Following ET, the catheter should be examined under the microscope to ensure that all embryos have been expelled.

If any embryos are retained in the catheter, they can be reloaded and transferred; it is unclear whether this impacts pregnancy rates.

The plunger on the syringe must remain completely engaged after ET so that negative pressure does not cause the embryos to be removed along with the catheter.

The embryo recipient may rest in the supine position for about 15-30 minutes; however, there is no evidence to support the benefit of this vs. immediate ambulation or for the use of a fibrin sealant with ET.

There are no good data to suggest that normal activities should be avoided after this time interval.

However, it may be prudent to avoid intercourse, or other activities that cause uterine contractions, for some days after the transfer.

If this was a fresh IVF cycle, there is usually an ongoing ovarian enlargement that indicates precautions against activities that may cause ovarian torsion.

There are no good studies to suggest which activities should be restricted during this time.

However, common sense suggests that contact sports and vigorous lifting or twisting should be avoided.

Post-Transfer Luteal Support

Luteal phase hormonal support is indicated following ET for a number of reasons.

The use of gonadotropin agonists and antagonists for ovarian stimulation suppresses natural endogenous LH production.

Oocyte retrieval may also mechanically disrupt ovarian corpus luteum development.

All of this results in inadequate luteal function to develop a receptive endometrium for preembryo implantation and for support of early pregnancy.

Luteal support is traditionally continued from day of oocyte retrieval until 8-10 weeks' gestation.

It may be possible to discontinue this earlier, especially if serum progesterone levels on the day of the pregnancy test are high.

Options for luteal support include the following:

– Progesterone vaginal cream or tablet (100-600 mg daily).

– Progesterone injection (25-50 mg daily, intramuscularly).

– Progesterone oral capsule (300-800 mg daily).

– Supplemental hCG (1,500–5,000 IU intramuscularly every 3 days).

– Progesterone vaginal 8% gel (90 mg daily).

Some evidence suggests that progesterone should be favored over hCG; it should be noted that hCG has a higher risk of OHSS.

New studies suggest that 8% vaginal progesterone gel and natural progesterone dissolving vaginal tablets (100 mg two times a day – to three times a day) may be equally efficacious.

There has been a vogue to consider the use of low dose aspirin as a potential means to improve implantation rates; however recent systematic reviews have failed to demonstrate any benefit.

RISKS OF IVF

Certain risks are associated with IVF:

– There is increasing evidence of a small increase in major birth defects, including septal heart defects and cleft lip.

– Multiple gestations carry significant risks, including preterm birth and increased maternal and fetal morbidity.

– Singleton and twin infants may have lower birthweights and earlier deliveries compared with naturally-conceived pregnancies, although the clinical significance of this is unclear.

– If a woman develops OHSS, there are risks for ascites, pleural effusion, renal dysfunction, blood clotting and even death; women may require hospitalization for pain control and fluid management, or paracentesis to remove excess peritoneal fluid; cycle cancellation may also be needed.

– Ovarian torsion, in which the ovary twists and cuts off its own blood supply, can also occur, especially with co-existing OHSS; symptoms include severe pain and tenderness in the lower abdomen, nausea and vomiting.

– Risks and complications of the actual oocyte retrieval procedure is very small, less than 1%; these include: infection, damage to bowel, bladder, vasculature, failure to retrieve any oocytes, inability to access the ovaries, intra-ovarian / peritoneal bleeding, and risks of anesthesia.

OVARIAN HYPERSTIMULATION SYNDROME

Introduction

Ovarian hyperstimulation syndrome (OHSS) is a serious and life-threatening iatrogenic complication of ovarian stimulation and ART.

The syndrome is characterized by ovarian enlargement and a shift of fluid from the intravascular to the extravascular space due to increased capillary permeability and ovarian neoangiogenesis.

This leads to accumulation of fluid in the peritoneal, pleural and, rarely, the pericardial cavities, resulting in intravascular fluid depletion and hemoconcentration.

Any woman undergoing ovarian stimulation is at risk; however, OHSS occurs more frequently in women with PCOS.

Women with high estradiol levels and/or a large number of follicles during ovulation induction have an increased risk of OHSS.

Its occurrence is dependent on the administration of hCG, and is extremely rare without hCG administration.

The incidence of OHSS is between 0.25% and 4% and severe hyperstimulation is seen in about one in 200 patients.

Pathophysiology of OHSS

During the last 10 years the pathophysiology of the syndrome has been extensively investigated.

The process is related to increased vascular permeability in the region surrounding the ovaries and their vasculature.

The crux is equilibrium between proangiogenic and antiangiogenic factors present in follicular fluid.

B-hCG and its analogs, estrogen, estradiol, prolactin, histamine and prostaglandins have all been implicated in OHSS.

Vascular endothelial growth factor (VEGF) plays a central role in the cascade of events leading to OHSS.

The renin-angiotensin-aldosterone system, LH, histamine, prostaglandins or ovarian prorenin may also have a role in the pathophysiology of OHSS.

Classification of OHSS

Mild OHSS:

−Abdominal distension.

−Mild pain.

−Ovarian size usually <8 cm.

Moderate OHSS:

−Features of mild OHSS and ultrasound evidence of ascites.

−Nausea, vomiting and diarrhea.

−Ovarian size usually 8-12 cm.

Severe OHSS:

- Clinical ascites and/or hydrothorax.

- Hemoconcentration (hematocrit > 45%, WBC >15000/mL).

- Coagulation and/or electrolyte disturbances

- Hypovolemia.

- Oliguria with elevated serum creatinine.

- Renal failure.

- Thromboembolic phenomena.

- Ovarian enlargement >12 cm.

A modification of this classification was proposed, allowing the identification of those women who require immediate hospitalization and differentiates between severe and life-threatening OHSS.

It also allows a simple comparison between different series reported in the literature.

The mild degree of OHSS is omitted because it is so common after ovarian stimulation for ART and does not require medical intervention.

Ultrasound evidence of ascites is maintained as part of moderate OHSS.

The presence of any abnormality in hepatic or renal functions would indicate Grade B severe OHSS.

Grade C includes women with respiratory syndrome, venous thromboembolism or renal shutdown – all medical emergencies that require intensive medical care.

Prediction of OHSS

Current management of OHSS relies on the prediction and active prevention.

Any patient undergoing ovarian stimulation is at risk of OHSS but it appears to be more frequent in younger women (aged <35 years) and women with PCOS, and is increased with exogenous hCG administration in the luteal phase or in conception cycles.

The majority of cases can be predicted by the combined use of ultrasound and endocrine monitoring.

Risk factors of OHSS:

– Young women (<35 years).

– PCOS.

– High and rapid rise of serum estradiol.

– Large number of follicles with a high portion of small and intermediate follicles.

– PCOS pattern for response to GnRH before hMG.

– Conception cycles, particularly multiple pregnancies.

– OHSS in a previous cycle.

- GnRH agonist use.

- Luteal phase supplementation with hCG.

- Multiple pregnancy.

Estradiol Monitoring

The estradiol level, above which different authors have recommended withholding hCG, has gradually increased.

There is general agreement that permissible levels are higher in ART cycles compared to in vivo conception.

Generally, the higher the serum estradiol and the quicker the rise, the higher the chance of OHSS.

In case where estradiol was >6000 pg/mL (approx. 20.000 nmol/L) there is a greater chance of developing severe OHSS.

There is general consensus that the chances of OHSS are minimal if estradiol is <1500 pg/mL.

Severe OHSS was reported in women with hypogonadotrophic hypogonadism during ovulation induction with urinary human FSH and hCG in the presence of low estradiol.

The development of severe OHSS in the presence of low estradiol levels is the exception rather than the rule.

However, it does demonstrate that estradiol is not the mediator of increased capillary permeability.

<u>Ultrasonographic Monitoring</u>

A correlation between the number and size of periovulatory follicles was observed by transvaginal ultrasonography and the development of OHSS.

The follicles were classified as small (5-8 mm), medium (9-15 mm) and large (16-25 mm).

A decrease in the fraction of mature follicles and an increase in the fraction of the very small follicles were associated with an increased risk of OHSS.

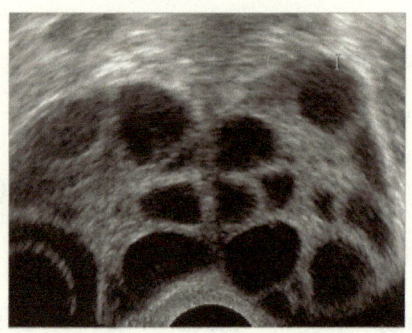

OHSS Ultrasound

Prevention of OHSS

There are numerous strategies for reducing the risk of OHSS, and the list is ever increasing:

<u>Withholding hCG</u>

Withholding hCG and cancellation of the IVF cycle has been the classic approach to reduce the risk of severe OHSS.

This creates a frustrating situation for both the physician and patient.

Reducing the Dose of hCG

There are very few data comparing the dose of hCG and the incidence of OHSS.

Three doses of hCG were compared to trigger ovulation (2000 IU; 5000 IU; 10.000 IU).

The number of oocytes was significantly lower when 2000 IU were used; a similar oocyte retrieval rate was achieved with 5000 and 10.000 IU with significantly less OHSS when 5000 IU was used.

Delaying hCG/Coasting

Delaying hCG or coasting has been used successfully to reduce the severity of OHSS.

OHSS was completely avoided by delaying hCG in 12 "overstimulated" women.

hMG was withheld for several days and hCG was administered when the leading follicles were 17-22 mm diameter.

During the withholding phase, follicular growth continued in all women, while estradiol levels declined in all but three and these three women conceived; ovulation was observed in six additional women.

The results of 40 IVF cycles in 32 women with PCOS were reported; the women were considered at risk of OHSS when estradiol levels were 1500 pg/mL.

Coasting significantly reduced the severity of OHSS; the clinical pregnancy rate was 20% and multiple pregnancy rate 50%, with severe OHSS in 2.5%.

The data of 17 women whose estradiol level rose above 6000 pg/mL and developed more than 30 follicles during COH for IVF was reported.

Coasting was continued for four to nine days until estradiol levels dropped to <3000 pg/mL; none of the women developed severe OHSS and 16 conceived.

GnRH Agonists to Trigger Ovulation

In a prospective randomized study of 179 women undergoing IVF, Leuprorelide acetate 500 µg or hCG 5000 IU was administered 34-36 hours before oocyte retrieval, with similar pregnancy rates in both groups.

Luteal phase estradiol and progesterone levels were significantly lower in the GnRH agonist group compared with the hCG group, and it was suggested that this may be beneficial in preventing OHSS.

The effectiveness of GnRH agonist to trigger ovulation has been studied in both uncontrolled and controlled studies.

In uncontrolled studies, the GnRH agonist was successful in triggering ovulation in 88% of the cases resulting in LH surge in 99% of cases compared to 98% with hCG and the pregnancy rate was 22% versus 17% (P <0.05).

In controlled studies where GnRH agonist was used to trigger ovulation, the incidence of OHSS was 0.9% (3/334).

GnRH Antagonist Protocol

The differential action of GnRH antagonists at both pituitary and ovarian receptors suggests that antagonist-suppressed cycles might result in a lower incidence of OHSS compared with agonist cycles.

A Cochrane review demonstrated that the incidence of severe OHSS was significantly lower in an antagonist protocol than in an agonist protocol.

Progesterone for Luteal Phase Support

The use of hCG in luteal phase support has been shown to confer significant benefits over placebo in agonist suppressed cycles; however, hCG is also known to increase the risk of OHSS.

The use of progestogens appears to halve this risk, while demonstrating similar improvements in pregnancy and miscarriage rates.

Cryopreservation of Embryos

Instead of canceling the cycle, it is also possible to administer hCG to retrieve the ocytes and to freeze all embryos; this does not exclude the risk for the early form of OHSS.

The removal of a large number of granulose cells from the follicles probably also decreases the risk.

In-Vitro Maturation (IVM)

In patients at high risk of developing OHSS, IVM of oocytes offers great potential for OHSS prevention.

Despite safety advantages, IVM is not yet widely used owing to a reduced live-birth rate in comparison with standard IVF.

Intravenous Albumin Administration

Intravenous albumin administration at the time of oocyte collection has been shown to have a preventive effect in cycles with a severe risk for OHSS.

However, a more recent prospective randomized trial of 488 cases in each arm seems to prove the inefficiency of human albumin.

Albumin administration also has side effects like viral transmission, nausea, vomiting, and febrile and allergic reactions.

Some authors have tested the effect of safer non-biological substitute (hydroxyethyl starch solution) with comparable physiological properties.

Insulin-Sensitizing Agents

A meta-analysis of eight randomized controlled trials of metformin co-administration during gonadotropin ovulation induction or IVF in women with PCOS found little benefit of metformin treatment in terms of improved ovulation or clinical outcome in this population but did note a significant positive effect on the incidence of OHSS.

Dopamine Agonist Administration

Cabergoline inhibits partially the VEGF receptor 2 phosphorylation levels and associated vascular permeability without affecting luteal angiogenesis and reduces the early onset of OHSS.

Treatment of OHSS

Mild OHSS

Mild ovarian hyperstimulation can develop into moderate or severe disease, especially if conception ensues.

Therefore, women with mild disease should be observed for enlarging abdominal girth, acute weight gain, and abdominal discomfort on an ambulatory basis for at least 2 weeks or until menstrual bleeding occurs.

Moderate OHSS

Treatment of moderate OHSS consists of observation, bed rest, provision of adequate fluids and sonographic monitoring of the size of cysts.

Serum electrolyte concentrations, hematocrits and creatinine levels should also be evaluated.

The beginning of the resolution of OHSS is apparent when the cysts shrink, as seen on two consecutive ultrasonographic examinations, and when clinical symptoms recede.

In contrast, early detection of progression to the severe form of the syndrome is marked by continuous weight gain (>2 lb/d), increased severity of existing symptoms, or appearance of new symptoms.

Severe OHSS

Severe form of OHSS is potentially lethal disorder; medical treatment is directed at maintaining intravascular blood volume.

Simultaneous goals are correcting the disturbed fluid and electrolyte balance, relieving secondary complications of ascites and hydrothorax and preventing thromboembolic phenomena.

If urine output is unsatisfactory, hyperosmolar intravenous therapy is indicated with an infusion of 200 mL of 25% human albumin.

The use of diuretics in patients with low urine production and hypovolemia is counterproductive and dangerous.

To prevent thrombosis, subcutaneous heparin 5000-7500 U/d is begun on the first day of admission; it is stopped after adequate mobilization.

To manage ascites, ultrasonographic-guided paracentesis is indicated if the patient has severe discomfort or pulmonary or renal compromise.

Intensive medical care may be needed in critical cases, such as renal failure, hepatic damage, thromboembolic phenomena, respiratory syndrome and multiorgan failure.

Surgery is necessary only in extreme cases, such as in the case of a ruptured cyst, ovarian torsion or internal hemorrhage.

Prognosis

– In mild or moderate OHSS, the prognosis is usually excellent.

– In severe OHSS, the prognosis is optimistic if good treatment is given.

FACTORS AFFECTING IVF OUTCOME

Thirty years after the birth of the first infant after IVF, the number of children born worldwide as a result of IVF already exceeds three million.

Clinical and laboratory procedures have been constantly improving and nowadays pregnancy rates of about 30% per transfer are routinely reported.

IVF is therefore an important method for correcting unfavorable demographic indices despite associated costs, being as high as one quarter of annual household expenditure in some countries.

Initially, IVF was performed in a natural cycle; since only one oocyte was collected at a time, the success rate was very low, with a live birth rate (LBR) of only 9.6%.

Treatment was also limited only to women with spontaneous ovulation.

The introduction of ovarian stimulation in 1981, first using CC and later gonadotropins and GnRH agonists increased the number of collected oocytes and embryos available for transfer.

At the same time, indications for IVF treatment broadened to anovulation of different etiologies.

Later on, ICSI allowed severe male reproductive disorders to be treated as well.

Initially, the simultaneous transfer of several embryos was favored because of the low chance of implantation.

In 1991, three embryos were transferred in 40.5% and more than 3 embryos in 24.6% of cycles, but the overall LBR per started cycle was only 12%.

The high multiple pregnancy rate has exposed a large number of children to health risks.

Compared with singleton births, perinatal mortality rates are at least four-fold higher for twins and at least six-fold higher for triplets.

Twins born after IVF have almost a ten-fold higher risk of being born prematurely than IVF singletons, and because of this a 3.8-fold increased risk of admittance to a neonatal intensive care unit.

There is accumulating evidence that if several embryos are created and one of them is selected for transfer on the basis of good morphology, pregnancy rate (PR) and LBR are high.

All other good quality embryos can be frozen and transferred later; this strategy results in a cumulative PR of up to 60% in young women.

Currently, elective single ET (eSET) is the recommended strategy in both Europe and U.S., but clinical practice shows little adherence to the guidelines outside the Nordic countries.

Traditionally, IVF outcome has been expressed in terms of biochemical or clinical pregnancies and total live births.

However, these parameters also include multiple gestations and births, which are considered to be complications of IVF because of the dimensions of their prematurity-related problems.

This is why a lengthy discussion on the definition of the main outcome of IVF treatment ended without reaching consensus.

Embryo Quality

The assessment of embryo quality in IVF is essential and it determines the number of embryos to be transferred and frozen.

Cleavage speed and degree of fragmentation were the first parameters to be assessed.

Other morphological aspects found to be related to embryo quality were cytoplasm appearance, blastomere irregularity and degree of fragmentation.

Together with cleavage rate, these factors were evaluated in the first embryo quality scoring method (the cumulative embryo score) which was aimed at optimizing PR while avoiding triplet and other higher-order pregnancies.

At present, morphological evaluation of the embryo routinely includes zona pellucida assessment, as a thick zona pellucida has been found to affect fertilization negatively.

Multinucleation of blastomeres is another factor that diminishes the chance of pregnancy.

Embryo quality is expressed not only in terms of morphology and cleavage speed two or three days after fertilization but also as regards the time of the first mitotic division.

Embryos which complete the first mitotic division within 25-27 h after insemination have been associated with higher PR (40.5% vs. 31.3%), compared with late-cleaving ones.

Embryo grading cannot give an accurate prediction of pregnancy; this is why evaluation of clinical factors helps predict outcome of IVF.

The majority of these factors are characteristics of the female rather than the male patient.

This can be explained by the fact that although the zygote contains equal amounts of chromosomal DNA of maternal and paternal origin, most of the cytoplasm and all the mitochondria originate from the oocyte.

The results of several studies have indicated a relationship between oocyte and embryo quality, but the importance for early embryo development of factors related to spermatozoa is less clear.

An analysis of cycles with shared oocytes in an oocyte donation program revealed that embryo morphology (blastomere uniformity and fragmentation) is determined by oocyte quality, while the cleavage rate is affected by both oocyte and spermatozoa quality.

Endometrial Receptivity

It has been estimated that uterine receptivity accounts for about 31-64% of implantation.

A blastocyst can implant into the endometrium only during a short period of time called the window of implantation.

It is believed that it lasts about 48 hours, beginning 6-10 days after the LH surge in a spontaneous cycle.

Embryo implantation is regulated by a multitude of factors; glycodelin is the major component of endometrial secretion and its expression is regulated by progesterone.

It is believed that the appearance of glycodelin secretion reflects endometrial maturation, which is essential for embryo implantation.

Glycodelin has immunosuppressive properties and contributes to the maintenance of pregnancy during the first trimester.

Accordingly, concentrations of serum glycodelin have been found to be decreased in women with early pregnancy loss.

It is believed that the outcome of the first few days after implantation is determined by embryo morphology but that the continuation of pregnancy beyond 6 weeks is more dependent on the combination of embryonic and uterine factors.

In humans, there is accumulating evidence of a molecular dialogue between the developing embryo and the maternal endometrial epithelium.

This crosstalk involves, among other things, nutrition markers such as leptin as well as factors regulated by insulin, such as IGFBP-1 and $\alpha v\beta 3$ integrin.

Female Age

The deleterious effect of increasing age on the outcome of IVF is indisputable.

Lower numbers of oocytes are collected and fewer embryos are created, leading to lower PR and LBR and increased miscarriage rate (MR).

It is generally considered that this decline starts after the age of 35 years and the effect is more pronounced after the age of 40.

Accordingly, female age is either studied in groups or in linear regression models.

Linear regression analysis of 1101 IVF cycles with ovum pickup showed a significant negative linear correlation between age and ongoing pregnancy rate.

The ongoing PR/ET declined from 26% in patients younger than 30 years of age to 9% in those aged 37 years, whereas the MR increased from 29% in women under the age of 40 to 50% in those ≥40 years old.

It is believed that women are born with a fixed number of oocytes arrested in the first meiotic division, and the numbers subsequently decline during their lives.

The number of germ cells reaches a maximum at mid-gestation during fetal life, and declines continuously thereafter.

This trend is accentuated at about the age of 37-38, when there is an acceleration of the loss of oogonia.

Exhaustion of the oocyte pool occurs around the age of 50 years, leading to menopause.

It has long been known that in spontaneous pregnancies the risk of chromosomal abnormalities increases with maternal age.

Likewise, studies of human oocytes have revealed a growing number of chromosomal abnormalities in the oocytes of older women.

As explained above, oocyte abnormalities are the main cause of embryonic chromosomal defects.

The occurrence of aneuploidy has been classically attributed to chromosomal non-disjunction during either meiosis I or II.

However, premature separation of chromatids during meiosis might be the main factor contributing to the formation of oocytes with abnormal chromosomal complements.

This is caused by the gradual but constant age-related degradation of cohesins and other factors holding the four chromatids together during metaphase I.

Human oocytes enter the first stage of meiosis during fetal life but are selected for further development years later in adult life.

Until then, the oocyte's mitochondria are exposed to reactive oxygen species (ROS), which damage the mitochondrial DNA.

This leads to abnormal oxidative metabolism and production of adenosine triphosphate, which might be responsible for abnormalities in the meiotic spindle.

The decline in fertility in older women can also be explained by telomere shortening due to the combined effects of prolonged exposure to ROS and telomerase deficiency.

Telomeres are repetitive DNA sequences at chromosomal ends; adequate telomere length is essential for the proper alignment of chromosomes during metaphase.

However this length might be diminished in oocytes from older women because of damage caused by ROS.

The enzyme telomerase protects against telomere shortening; its activity in female germ cells is significant during early fetal life but is limited in later-stage oocytes.

The increased incidence of oocyte abnormalities with maternal age can also be explained by hormonal imbalances, abnormalities in follicular development due to ageing of the somatic cells surrounding the oocyte and impaired perifollicular microcirculation.

Low Ovarian Response

Low response is observed when the outcome of ovarian stimulation is suboptimal, leading to a low chance of pregnancy and birth after IVF.

Low response is one of the significant problems of IVF because it occurs in up to 24% of cases.

The diagnosis, prognostic factors and treatment options for women with low response have been the subject of several reviews.

Although much is known about the nature of low response, numerous definitions exist because of the different diagnostic tools used in evaluation of the infertile patient.

They include the following:

−Female age ≥40 years.

−Elevated day 3 FSH (≥7 to ≥15 mIU/mL).

−Estradiol level <200 pg/mL on day 5 of stimulation.

−Low peak estradiol level during stimulation (<300 to <500 pg/mL).

−Low number of growing follicles (from <3 to <5 on day of hCG).

−Low number of collected oocytes (<3 to <5).

−Lately, the definition of poor response also includes poor embryo quality.

Body Mass Index (BMI)

Even though the consequences of obesity in women are well known, in IVF there is controversy regarding the effect of obesity on the outcome of treatment.

Obese women require higher gonadotropin doses for ovarian stimulation, despite which, fewer oocytes are collected; however, similar numbers have also been reported.

In a study of 3600 IVF cycles, an elevated BMI was found to be associated with decreased cumulative PR after controlling for multiple confounding factors.

Overweight women had only an 80% chance, obese only a 70% chance and very obese women only a 50% chance of pregnancy compared with women of normal weight, even after several IVF cycles.

Obesity also diminishes cumulative LBR; it was estimated that because of a lower success rate at every step of IVF, only 17% of obese patients have a live birth, compared with 21% of normal-weight women.

Despite this evidence, it is difficult to draw final conclusions about the effect of obesity on the outcome of IVF because of the contradictory results of miscarriage studies.

Polycystic Ovary Syndrome (PCOS)

PCOS is the most common endocrine disorder in women of reproductive age.

According to the Rotterdam consensus, it is diagnosed when two of the three following criteria are present:

– Oligo/anovulation,

– Clinical and/or biochemical signs of hyperandrogenemia, and

– Polycystic ovaries ($\geq$12 follicles measuring 2-9 mm in each ovary).

The etiology of PCOS is unknown; insulin resistance is a main feature of the pathogenesis of the syndrome.

Obesity, especially the abdominal type, is another characteristic of PCOS; obesity exacerbates endocrine disturbances of PCOS but even lean women with PCOS have fertility problems similar to those occurring in obese women without the syndrome.

In IVF, PCOS is a known risk factor of OHSS, a rare but serious complication of ovarian stimulation.

More oocytes are usually collected from women with PCOS compared with subjects without the syndrome.

However, PCOS has been associated with lower cumulative PR after IVF after controlling for obesity, age and other factors.

Earlier studies revealed an increased MR in these patients; however, more recent research has showed that PCOS loses its independent effect on miscarriage after controlling for obesity and a number of other factors.

Furthermore, it has been demonstrated that insulin resistance increases the risk of miscarriage independently of BMI or PCOS status.

Other Factors

Women with tubal factor infertility have been found to have lower LBR and lower cumulative LBR.

Male factor infertility and endometriosis have also been associated with a low chance of live birth.

Other factors with an effect on the outcome of IVF are smoking, primary infertility, a long duration of infertility and a high number of previous IVF treatments.

IVF-RELATED TECHNIQUES

INTRACYTOPLASMIC SPERM INJECTION (ICSI)

ICSI is a micromanipulation procedure in which a single sperm is injected directly into the cytoplasm of the oocyte.

The first successful pregnancies after ICSI were reported in 1992 and today it is used in over 60% of the SART reported IVF cases.

Indications

ICSI has traditionally been applied in cases of male factor infertility, (such as grossly abnormal semen parameters or low sperm concentration), and in cases using sperm surgically retrieved from the epididymis or testis.

Use of ICSI has expanded over the years and now is often used in cases in which there are very few oocytes to work with, in some cases of PGD such as those involving removal of the polar body, and to avoid sperm contamination in PGD cases in which PCR is used.

ICSI also often used for patients who have failed fertilization in previous IVF attempts and for couples with unexplained infertility to avoid the possibility of failed fertilization.

Technique

Various sperm preparation techniques are available for ICSI, depending on the quality of the available sample.

In many cases a simple wash or swim-up technique is suitable; in cases using a surgically retrieved tissue sample, the sample is processed and the sperm retrieved.

Sperm are often chosen based on morphological characteristics including shape, light reaction, and motion patterns.

Once a single sperm is chosen, it is immobilized by breaking the tail at the mid piece with a glass pipette.

This immobilization step is thought to release sperm cytosolic components thought to be important for oocyte activation and fertilization.

After retrieval, oocytes are incubated for 3-4 hours prior to preparation for ICSI.

After incubation, the cumulus cells are removed from the oocyte and the oocyte is observed for maturational status.

Oocytes that are mature (that is, have extruded the first polar body) are injected directly with the immobilized sperm.

For ICSI, the immobilized sperm is aspirated tail first into an injection pipette and the oocyte held in place on a holding pipette with a small amount of suction.

The oocyte is held by the holding pipette such that the polar body is at 6 or 12 o'clock, which helps avoid damage to the meiotic spindle.

The injection pipette is advanced into the cytoplasm of the oocyte and the sperm cell is slowly deposited.

Injected oocytes are incubated and observed for subsequent fertilization 12-17 hours after injection.

Risks

ICSI has been associated with several risks for the offspring, including increased risks of transmitted chromosomal aberrations and new, spontaneous chromosomal aberrations that are most often abnormalities of the sex chromosomes.

Also, the process of stripping the cumulus from the oocyte can be vigorous, and in some cases this procedure can result in damage to the oocytes.

Because of these risks, it is not recommended that ICSI be universally applied to all IVF cases although its use is increasingly common.

The incidence of chromosomal abnormalities is higher among subfertile men, and thus some of the increased incidence of chromosomal abnormalities has been attributed to subfertile men passing on the abnormalities.

There does not appear to be any increased risk of congenital malformations or epigenetic disorders among children born after ICSI, although long-term follow up of these children is needed.

Success

Typical ICSI fertilization rates range in different studies anywhere between 60 and 75%.

Fertilization success with ICSI may be lower with surgically retrieved sperm than with ejaculated sperm, but these rates are typically still acceptable.

Fertilization rates with cryopreserved sperm appear to be equivalent to those seen with fresh sperm.

Pregnancy and delivery rates with embryos resulting after ICSI fertilization fare just as well as those achieved with embryos resulting from conventional insemination.

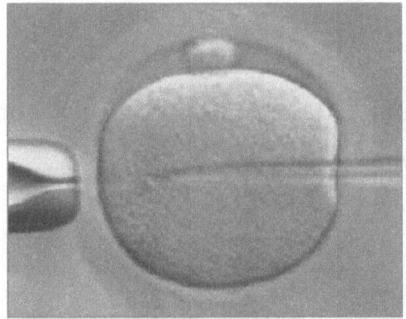

Intracytoplasmic Sperm Injection (ICSI)

GAMETE INTRAFALLOPIAN TRANSFER (GIFT)

The first successful report of GIFT resulting in a live birth was in 1979.

GIFT is performed today in less than 1% of ART procedures.

Indications

The main indications for this procedure include patients requiring ART where resources for IVF are not available, and patients who are opposed to IVF for religious or other personal reasons.

Technique

In GIFT, a patient undergoes laparoscopic oocyte retrieval in a natural cycle or after COH with CC or gonadotropins.

Once the oocytes are retrieved, they are placed into the fimbriated end of the fallopian tube along with prepared sperm.

Risks

The major risks associated with GIFT include the risks associated with anesthesia, whether epidural or general anesthesia, and the risks of laparoscopic surgery.

While the chances of problems arising with these components of GIFT are low, they are still greater than those risks associated with standard IVF procedures with uterine ET.

Advantages

The benefits of GIFT over IVF are that GIFT does not require an IVF lab or IVF technical expertise, which makes it an attractive option for people without access to these resources.

Disadvantages

The disadvantage of GIFT is that it does not allow one to determine if fertilization of the oocytes has taken place, or evaluation of embryonic development.

Also, GIFT requires that at least one fallopian tube be patent, and the necessary components of the treatment are much more time consuming than the components required for standard IVF.

Success

If patients are properly chosen, the chances of successful pregnancy with GIFT are similar to those of standard IVF.

ZYGOTE INTRAFALLOPIAN TRANSFER (ZIFT)

Similar to GIFT, ZIFT involves the direct transfer of reproductive tissue into the fallopian tubes;

Unlike GIFT, the transferred tissue is a zygote.

ZIFT accounts for less than 1% of ART procedures performed in the U.S. each year.

Indications

One established indication for the application of ZIFT is when the woman's cervix has an anatomical abnormality or has been damaged by surgery or irradiation such that the ET catheter cannot be passed through the cervix.

Technique

In ZIFT, cultured zygotes are transferred directly into the fallopian tubes via laparoscopy.

Risks

Similar to GIFT, ZIFT procedure poses certain risks to patients; major risks include those associated with anesthesia and laparoscopy.

Advantages

The greatest advantage of using ZIFT rather than GIFT is that ZIFT allows a determination of whether or not oocytes fertilize and the quality of the resulting embryos.

Disadvantages

Disadvantages include extra work, facilities, and expenses associated with embryo culture; at least 1 patent fallopian tube required; operating room time and patient recovery.

Success

In properly chosen patients, ZIFT pregnancy and delivery rates are comparable to those seen in IVF.

EMBRYO CRYOPRESERVATION

Embryo cryopreservation is the process of freezing embryos for future use.

The first child born after embryo freezing, correctly termed cryopreservation, was born in 1984.

Today, approximately 25% of children born using ART have developed from cryopreserved embryos.

Indications

Embryo cryopreservation is a cost-effective strategy for increasing cumulative pregnancy rates in IVF cycles when fresh embryos are transferred in the first cycle; it is an essential component of elective single ET programs.

Cumulative pregnancy rates using elective single ET, coupled with subsequent transfer of cryopreserved embryos, have been shown to be equal to pregnancy rates seen in cycles in which multiple embryos are transferred.

The benefits of this strategy include decreased risk of multiple gestations and decreased overall costs when taking into consideration the expenses associated with multiple gestations.

Embryo cryopreservation has been applied effectively in women undergoing COH who develop OHSS.

In such cases, viable embryos can be frozen and transferred back at a later time when the OHSS symptoms have subsided.

Finally, embryo banking via embryo cryopreservation is an established practice for women facing gonadotoxic therapy, such as radiation or chemotherapy, who desire fertility preservation.

Technique

Protocols and practices for embryo cryopreservation vary widely among programs offering assisted reproductive technologies.

The two methods widely used to freeze embryos include slow freeze and vitrification.

Slow freezing has long been the preferred method of embryo cryopreservation; however, vitrification is becoming more common.

The main goal of both methods is to reduce the formation of intracellular ice during the cryopreservation process, as it can lead to damage and developmental arrest of the embryonic cells.

Slow freezing does this by cooling the embryo and its surrounding environment at a controlled rate in the presence of a low concentration of cryoprotectants.

In vitrification protocols, the cell and the surrounding solution are directly solidified to a glass-like state without forming ice crystals.

This process requires high concentrations of cryoprotectants and rapid cooling rates provided by directly plunging the embryos into liquid nitrogen.

Vitrification offers several potential advantages over slow-freeze protocols, as it is a faster, easier, less costly process.

The major concern over vitrification is the high concentration of cryoprotectants required.

Several studies suggest vitrification may offer improved survival of embryos after thawing.

However, long-term data, including pregnancy outcomes, are needed to determine which method is optimal, and these results may vary from center to center depending on the experience of the staff in the IVF laboratory.

Timing the thawing and transfer of cryopreserved embryos depends on the developmental stage of the embryos when they were frozen.

Most programs freeze embryos at one of the following three developmental stages:

– Zygote (2 days following insemination of oocytes),

– Cleavage stage (3 days after insemination of oocytes), and

– Blastocyst stage (day 5 or 6 following insemination of oocytes).

There are advantages and disadvantages to freezing embryos at any of these time points.

Freezing embryos at the zygote stage often yields better survival rates after thawing of the embryos.

However, it does not allow for ample morphologic information from the embryo to discern which embryos are to be transferred and which embryos are to be frozen.

Therefore, freezing embryos at the zygote stage is ideal for patients planning on freezing all of their embryos and not planning to undergo fresh ET.

Alternatively, freezing embryos at the blastocyst stage may decrease the chances of embryo survival, as the fluid in the blastocoels is at risk for ice-crystal formation.

On the other hand, freezing at the blastocyst stage also allows for improved selection from embryos available for fresh transfer, as blastocysts yield more morphological data than embryos at the other stages of development.

Programs often develop preferences for embryo stage at freezing based on the clinical scenario and their laboratory's experience.

It is important to note that it is not possible to select the embryos most likely to result in a viable child on morphological features alone.

Various protocols exist for transfer of cryopreserved embryos:

Natural Cycle ET

Natural cycle protocols for cryopreserved ET involve transfer of thawed embryos at the appropriate time during a natural menstrual cycle based on timing of the LH surge.

For example, a thawed blastocyst would be thawed 4 days after a woman's natural LH surge and transferred on the 5th day, the time when the uterus would be expected to be receptive for implantation of a blastocyst.

Progesterone supplementation may be used in natural cycle protocols, although endogenous luteal progesterone production after the LH surge should be sufficient to support pregnancy.

Artificial Cycle ET

Protocols involving hormonal supplementation are available to artificially prepare the endometrium for transfer of thawed cryopreserved embryos.

These protocols may or may not utilize a GnRH agonist such as leuprolide to suppress the pituitary-ovarian axis.

Regardless, in artificial cycles, estrogen is initiated on cycle day one and gradually increased.

On about cycle day 15, serum progesterone and estrogen concentrations are assessed to ensure that follicular development and/or ovulation have not occurred.

If this is the case and the endometrial development is sufficient, progesterone supplementation is begun.

Again, transfer of embryos is timed based on developmental stage of the embryos when they were frozen.

Risks

In general, the cryopreservation process may damage embryos such that they are not viable or capable of resulting in a pregnancy.

Further, not all embryos survive the thawing process, so having cryopreserved embryos in storage does not guarantee a patient will be able to utilize them; this is important to discuss with patients.

Advantages

For patients who have embryos in storage, preparation for a frozen ET is less time consuming and labor intensive than preparation required for a fresh ET, and it is often less costly than cycles using fresh embryos.

Disadvantages

Frozen ET cycles may yield lower pregnancy rates than fresh ET cycles.

In fact, ASRM/SART guidelines recommend that regardless of whether embryos are fresh or frozen, the same number should be transferred to women depending on their age.

Success

Data from the SART, representing approximately 85% of U.S. ART centers, demonstrate lower live-birth rates after frozen ET, compared to fresh ET in women up to age 40.

The data representing women aged 41 and older are less clear, as it appears live-birth rates may be comparable and perhaps even higher in women receiving frozen embryos compared to those receiving fresh embryos.

What makes these data a bit more complicated is that it is not clear for the frozen embryo cycles whether the success rates are characteristic of the age of the women when the embryos were frozen, or when they were transferred.

Centers should use their own data when discussing pregnancy and live-birth rates using fresh versus frozen embryos.

ASSISTED HATCHING (AH)

Like ICSI, AH is another micromanipulation technique used in ART.

The first reported use of AH in human embryos was in 1990; this report demonstrated an increased implantation rate in embryos in which AH was performed.

Oocytes are surrounded by the zona pellucida - a structure with important roles in oocyte fertilization.

Once an oocyte is fertilized, the zona pellucida remains as a shell surrounding the resulting embryo.

The zona pellucida continues to be important as it is thought to play a role in early embryonic development.

At the blastocyst stage of embryonic development, the embryo must "hatch" from the zona pellucida in order for implantation to occur.

There is evidence that a thick or hardened zona pellucida can impair hatching, which subsequently could impede implantation.

Indications

There are several clinical scenarios in which AH is thought to be helpful.

These scenarios include those of previously failed implantation (that is, embryos transferred, but no evidence of implantation), women of advanced age, women with elevated FSH levels, embryos with thickened zonae, and use of cryopreserved embryos.

In these scenarios, the zona is generally thought to be thicker or tougher, and result in a more difficult hatching.

Technique

AH may be accomplished using several methods, including

- Laser-AH,
- AH with the application of an acidic solution, and
- Mechanical-AH in which a needle is used to make a slit in the zona pellucida.

Risks

Although AH is a relatively simple procedure to perform, it does pose potential risk for damage to the embryo.

AH has also been associated with a possible increase in the chances of multiple gestations - likely by improving implantation rates of embryos in cycles in which multiple embryos are transferred back.

If elective single ET were to be used, this would not be an issue, as it does not appear to increase the chances of monozygotic twinning.

Advantages

It may be worthwhile to perform AH in cycles for women who have previously failed to conceive with IVF, women of advanced age, women with elevated FSH levels, women using frozen embryos, and women whose embryos have a thickened zona pellucida.

Disadvantages

Aside from the potential risks that AH poses, the only other potential disadvantages are that AH can increase the laboratory time and equipment needs for performing an IVF cycle.

Success

The data to support the use of AH in all of the scenarios mentioned on the previous slide are not entirely clear.

A 2009 meta-analysis that incorporated data from multiple other smaller studies suggests AH may improve pregnancy rates in women undergoing IVF.

However, many of the included studies failed to report live birth as an outcome, and this is generally the most relevant outcome.

Live-birth rates did not appear to be improved by AH based on the studies that did include this outcome.

The discrepancies in different trials included in this study may be due to variations in hatching protocols (for example, laser-AH versus acid-AH), and different inclusion and exclusion criteria for study populations.

PREIMPLANTATION GENETIC DIAGNOSIS (PGD)

The term "preimplantation genetic testing" describes procedures involving the removal of a polar body from an oocyte, or one or more cells from an embryo (blastomeres or trophoectoderm cells) to test for mutations in gene sequence or aneuploidy before transfer.

The term "preimplantation genetic diagnosis" (PGD) applies when one or both genetic parents carry a gene mutation or a balanced chromosomal rearrangement and testing is performed to determine whether that specific mutation or an unbalanced chromosomal complement has been transmitted to the oocyte or embryo.

The term "preimplantation genetic screening" (PGS) applies when the genetic parents are known or presumed to be chromosomally normal and their embryos are screened for some abnormalities, commonly aneuploidy.

Indications

PGD is indicated for couples at risk for transmitting a specific genetic disease or abnormality to their offspring.

These include couples in which one partner is known to be carrying a single gene mutation, both partners are carriers of a single gene mutation, one partner has a balanced translocation, inversion or other structural rearrangement, or one partner is a mosaic or is carrying an abnormal karyotype but still has the potential for normal gametes.

Mosaicism occurs when an individual has two or more cell populations with a different chromosomal makeup.

Males with Klinefelter syndrome have at least one extra copy of the X chromosome in each cell.

Variants of Klinefelter syndrome involve more than one extra X chromosome or extra copies of both X and Y chromosomes in each cell.

PGD also can be performed and may be elected by patients who carry mutations such as BRCA-1 that do not cause a specific disease but are thought to confer significantly increased risk for a disease.

PGD also can be performed for sex selection to control the sex of offspring to achieve a desired sex

Technique

PGD is performed by removing a cell from the day-3 embryo, which usually has 6-8 cells. This cell, called a blastomere, is tested for the disorder of concern.

A hole is made by laser in the zona pellucida of the embryo at approximately the 3:00 position.

An AH micropipette containing medium is inserted into the hole in the zona pellucida, and medium is gently expelled into the embryo.

The blastomere is pushed out of the hole in the zona pellucida, where it is successfully isolated from the embryo.

For maternally inherited mutations, genetic analysis can be performed on the oocyte by removing the first and, sometimes, the second polar body and by inferring the genetic composition of the oocyte from the result.

There are two different techniques for PGD:

Polymerase Chain Reaction (PCR)

A single gene defect is usually studied by utilizing a PCR to amplify the numbers of copies including the mutation so it can be detected.

Primers are developed to surround the genetic mutation; the affected individual's white blood cells are tested to make sure that the mutation can be detected using the designed primers.

There are a few diseases that have specific mutations that do not need this pretesting.

Fluorescence In Situ Hybridization (FISH)

Balanced translocations, mosaicism, or aneuploidy are usually tested using FISH.

FISH helps identify where a particular gene falls within an individual's chromosomes by using DNA probes labeled with distinctly colored fluorochromes that bind to specific DNA sequences.

The number of fluorescent signals of a particular color reflects the number of copies of each of the chromosomal segments of interest.

The fixation and labeling are very sensitive, but this technique has multiple technical limitations.

Results

Results are usually available in about 2 days, but techniques are changing rapidly and results may soon be available more quickly.

Results of testing are:

– Affected,

– Unaffected, and

– No result or un-interpretable.

Embryos then are selected from the normal embryos at blastocyst stage for transfer.

Limitations

There are some significant limitations to the use of PGD. Only those embryos diagnosed as "not affected" can be transferred.

It should be noted that biopsied embryos tend to have slower growth than normal, and may not become blastocysts; thus there may not be embryos suitable for transfer.

The major challenges of PGD relate primarily to the relatively short interval of time available for analysis and the fact that only one or two cells can be analyzed (compared to the hundreds of cells obtained via amniocentesis or CVS); results may be conclusive, inconclusive, or false negative.

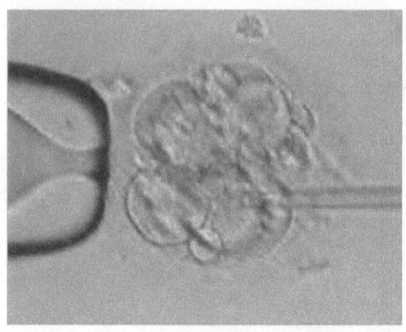 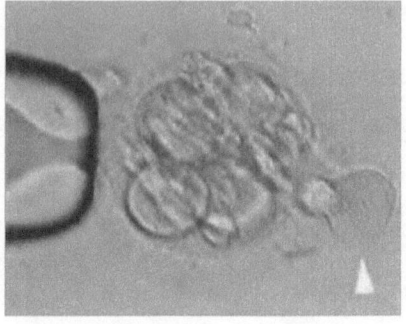

Preimplantation Genetic Diagnosis (PGD)

REFERENCES

– Abou-Setta A, Peters L, D'Angelo A, Sallam H, Hart R, Al-Inany H. Post-embryo transfer interventions for assisted reproduction technology cycles. Cochrane Database Syst Rev. 2014; 8: CD006567.

– Aghajanova L, Hamilton A, Giudice L. Uterine receptivity to human embryonic implantation: Histology, biomarkers, and transcriptomics. Semin Cell Dev Biol. 2008; 19: 201-11.

– Al-Inany H, Youssef M, Ayeleke R, Brown J, Lam W, Broekmans F. Gonadotrophin-releasing hormone antagonists for assisted reproductive technology. Cochrane Database Syst Rev. 2016; 4: CD001750.

– Allersma T, Farquhar C, Cantineau A. Natural cycle in vitro fertilisation (IVF) for subfertile couples. Cochrane Database Syst Rev. 2013; 8: CD010550.

– Armstrong S, Bhide P, Jordan V, Pacey A, Farquhar C. Time-lapse systems for embryo incubation and assessment in assisted reproduction. Cochrane Database Syst Rev. 2018; 5: CD011320.

– Baczkowski T, Kurzawa R, Glabowski W. Methods of embryo scoring in IVF. Reprod Biol. 2004; 4: 5-22.

– Balen A, St James. Assisted conception. In: Adam H Balen, editor. Infertility in practice, 3rd edition. Informa Healthcare; 2008.

– Bay B, Lyngsø J, Hohwü L, Kesmodel U. Childhood growth of singletons conceived following in vitro fertilisation or intracytoplasmic sperm injection: a systematic review and meta-analysis. BJOG. 2019; 126: 158-66.

– Bellver J, Melo M, Bosch E, Serra V, Remohí J, Pellicer A. Obesity and poor reproductive outcome: the potential role of the endometrium. Fertil Steril. 2007: 88: 446-51.

– Bellver J, Munoz E, Ballesteros A, Soares S, Bosch E, Simón C, et al. Intravenous albumin does not prevent moderate-severe OHSS in high-risk IVF patients: A randomized controlled study. Hum Reprod. 2003; 18: 2283-8.

– Bergh C. Single ET: a mini-review. Hum Reprod. 2005; 20: 323-7.

– Betts D, Madan P. Permanent embryo arrest: molecular and cellular concepts. Mol Hum Reprod. 2008; 14: 445-53.

– Boomsma C, Fauser B, Macklon N. Pregnancy complications in women with PCOS. Semin Reprod Med. 2008; 26: 72-84.

– Bosteels J, van Wessel S, Weyers S, Broekmans F, D'Hooghe T, Bongers M, et al. Hysteroscopy for treating subfertility associated with suspected major uterine cavity abnormalities. Cochrane Database Syst Rev. 2018; 12: CD009461.

– Broekmans F, Knauff E, te Velde E, Macklon N, Fauser B. Female reproductive ageing: current knowledge and future trends. Trends Endocrinol Metab. 2007; 18: 58-65.

– Broekmans F, Kwee J, Hendriks D, Mol B, Lambalk C. A systematic review of tests predicting ovarian reserve and IVF outcome. Hum Reprod Update. 2006; 12: 685-718.

– Caballero-Campo P, Dominguez F, Coloma J, Meseguer M, Remohi J, Pellicer A, et al. Hormonal and embryonic regulation of chemokines IL-8, MCP-1 and RANTES in the human endometrium during the window of implantation. Mol Hum Reprod. 2002; 8: 375-84.

– Carizza C, Abdelmassih V, Abdelmassih S, Ravizzini P, Salgueiro L, Salgueiro PT, et al. Cabergoline reduces the early onset of OHSS: A prospective randomized study. RBM Online. 2008; 17: 751-5.

– Carney S, Das S, Blake D, Farquhar C, Seif M, Nelson L. Assisted hatching on assisted conception (IVF/ICSI). Cochrane Database Syst Rev. 2012; 12: CD001894.

– Cissen M, Bensdorp A, Cohlen B, Repping S, de Bruin J, van Wely M. Assisted reproductive technologies for male subfertility. Cochrane Database Syst Rev. 2016; 2: CD000360.

– Collins J. An international survey of the health economics of IVF and ICSI. Hum Reprod Update. 2002; 8: 265-77.

– Costello M, Chapman M, Conway U. A systematic review and meta-analysis of randomized controlled trials on metformin co-administration during gonadotropin ovulation induction or IVF in women with PCOS. Hum Reprod. 2006; 21: 1387-99.

– Das S, Blake D, Farquhar C, Seif MM. Assisted hatching on assisted conception (IVF and ICSI). Cochrane Database Syst Rev. 2009; 2: CD001894.

– Daya S, Gunby J. Luteal phase support in assisted reproduction cycles. Cochrane Database Syst Rev. 2004; 3: CD004830.

– Daya S. GnRH agonist protocols for pituitary desensitization in IVF and GIFT cycles. Cochrane Database of Systematic Reviews 2000; 1: CD001299.

– Dechaud H, Anahory T, Reyftmann L, Loup V, Hamamah S, Hedon B. Obesity does not adversely affect results in patients who are undergoing IVF-ET. EJOGRB. 2006; 127: 88-93.

– Delvigne A, Rozenberg S. Epidemiology and prevention of OHSS: A review. Hum Reprod Update. 2002; 8: 559-77.

– Dickey R. The relative contribution of ARTs and ovulation induction to multiple births in the U.S. 5 years after the SART/ASRM recommendation to limit the number of embryos transferred. Fertil Steril. 2007; 88: 1554-61.

– Djahanbakhch O, Ezzati M, Zosmer A. Reproductive ageing in women. J Pathol. 2007; 211: 219-31.

- Ebner T, Yaman C, Moser M, Sommergruber M, Feichtinger O, Tews G. Prognostic value of first polar body morphology on fertilization rate and embryo quality in ICSI. Hum Reprod. 2000; 15: 427-30.

- Edwards R, Steptoe P. Current status of in-vitro fertilisation and implantation of human embryos. Lancet 1983; 2: 1265-9.

- El-Mazny A, Abou-Salem N, El-Sherbiny W, Saber W. Outpatient hysteroscopy: a routine investigation before ARTs? Fertil Steril. 2011; 95: 272-6.

- ESHRE Campus Course Report. Prevention of twin pregnancies after IVF/ICSI by single ET. Hum Reprod. 2001; 16: 790-800.

- Ethics Committee of the ASRM. Sex selection and preimplantation genetic diagnosis. Fertil Steril. 2004; 82: S245-8.

- European Orgalutran Study Group, Borm G, Mannaerts B. Treatment with the GnRH antagonist ganirelix in women undergoing COH with recombinant FSH is effective, safe and convenient: results of controlled, randomized, multicenter trial. Hum Reprod. 2000; 15: 1490-8.

- Farquhar C, Rombauts L, Kremer JA, Lethaby A, Ayeleke R. Oral contraceptive pill, progestogen or oestrogen pretreatment for ovarian stimulation protocols for women undergoing ARTs. Cochrane Database Syst Rev. 2017; 5: CD006109.

- Fedorcsák P, Dale P, Storeng R, Ertzeid G, Bjercke S, Oldereid N, et al. Impact of overweight and underweight on assisted reproduction treatment. Hum Reprod. 2004; 19: 2523-8.

- Ferraretti A, Gianaroli L, Magli M, Bafaro G, Colacurci N. Female poor responders. Mol Cell Endocrinol. 2000; 161: 59-66.

- Fisch JD, Keskintepe L, Sher G. GnRH agonist/antagonist conversion with estrogen priming in low responders with prior IVF failure. Fertil Steril. 2008; 89: 342-7.

– Gardner D. Evaluation and preparation of infertile couple for IVF. In: David R, editor. IVF a practical approach, 1st edition. Informa Healthcare; 2007.

– Ghobara T, Gelbaya T, Ayeleke R. Cycle regimens for frozen-thawed embryo transfer. Cochrane Database Syst Rev. 2017; 7: CD003414.

– Glujovsky D, Farquhar C, Quinteiro Retamar A, Alvarez Sedo C, Blake D. Cleavage stage versus blastocyst stage embryo transfer in assisted reproductive technology. Cochrane Database Syst Rev. 2016; 6: CD002118.

– Granne I, Child T, Hartshorne G; British Fertility Society. Embryo cryopreservation: evidence for practice. Hum Fertil (Camb). 2008; 11: 159-72.

– Guzick D, Overstreet J, Factor-Litvak P, Brazil C, Nakajima S, Coutifaris C et al. Sperm morphology, motility, and concentration in fertile and infertile men. National Cooperative Reproduction Medicine Network. N Engl J Med. 2001; 345: 1388-93.

– Harb H, Ghosh J, Al-Rshoud F, Karunakaran B, Gallos I, Coomarasamy A. Hydrosalpinx and pregnancy loss: a systematic review and meta-analysis. Reprod Biomed Online. 2019; 38: 427-41.

– Heijnen E, Eijkemans M, Hughes E, Laven J, Macklon N, Fauser B. A meta-analysis of outcomes of conventional IVF in women with PCOS. Hum Reprod Update. 2006; 12: 13-21.

– Henkel R, Schill W. Sperm preparation for ART. Reprod Biol Endocrinol. 2003; 1: 108.

– Isik A, Vicdan K. Combined approach as an effective method in the prevention of severe OHSS. EJOGRB. 2001; 97: 208-12.

– Johnson N, Mak W, Sowter M. Surgical treatment for tubal disease in women due to undergo IVF. Cochrane Database Syst Rev. 2001; 3: CD002125.

– Kamath M, Maheshwari A, Bhattacharya S, Lor K, Gibreel A. Oral medications including clomiphene citrate or aromatase inhibitors with gonadotropins for controlled ovarian stimulation in women undergoing in vitro fertilisation. Cochrane Database Syst Rev. 2017; 11: CD008528.

– Kligman I, Rosenwaks Z. Differentiating clinical profiles: predicting good responders, poor responders, and hyperresponders. Fertil Steril. 2001; 76: 1185-90.

– Klonoff-Cohen H, Bleha J, Lam-Kruglick P. A prospective study of the effects of female and male caffeine consumption on the reproductive endpoints of IVF and GIFT. Hum Reprod. 2002; 17: 1746-54.

– Klonoff-Cohen H, Lam-Kruglick P, Gonzalez C. Effects of maternal and paternal alcohol consumption on the success rates of IVF and GIFT. Fertil Steril. 2003; 79: 330-9.

– Kovacs G. IVF: indications, stimulation and clinical Techniques. in: James M, Mark L, editors. The subfertility handbook, 1st edition. Cambridge University Press; 1997.

– Kuivasaari P, Hippelainen M, Anttila M, Heinonen S. Effect of endometriosis on in vitro fertilisation (IVF) / intracytoplasmic sperm injection (ICSI) outcome: stage III/IV endometriosis worsens cumulative pregnancy and live-born rates. Hum Reprod. 2005; 20: 3130-5.

– Kwan I, Bhattacharya S, Kang A, Woolner A. Monitoring of stimulated cycles in assisted reproduction (IVF and ICSI). Cochrane Database Syst Rev. 2014; 8: CD005289.

– Lambers MJ, Mager E, Goutbeek J, McDonnell J, Homburg R, Schats R, et al. Factors determining early pregnancy loss in singleton and multiple implantations. Hum Reprod. 2007; 22: 275-9.

– Lensen S, Wilkinson J, Leijdekkers J, La Marca A, Mol B, Marjoribanks J, et al. Individualised gonadotropin dose selection using markers of ovarian reserve for women undergoing IVF/ICSI. Cochrane Database Syst Rev. 2018; 2: CD012693.

– Lintsen A, Pasker-de Jong P, de Boer E, Burger C, Jansen C, Braat D, et al. Effects of subfertility cause, smoking and body weight on the success rate of IVF. Hum Reprod. 2005; 20: 1867-75.

– Liu J, Aziz R, Dodson W, Fritz M, Van Voorhis B, editors. Précis – Reproductive Endocrinology, 3rd edition. Washington, DC: ACOG; 2007.

– Loh S, Wang J, Matthews C. The influence of BMI, basal FSH and age on the response to gonadotropin stimulation in non-PCOS patients. Hum Reprod. 2002; 17: 1207-11.

– Loutradi K, Kolibianakis E, Venetis C, Papanikolaou E, Pados G, Bontis I, et al. Cryopreservation of human embryos by vitrification or slow freezing: a systematic review and meta-analysis. Fertil Steril. 2008; 90: 186-93.

– Lundin K, Bergh C, Hardarson T. Early embryo cleavage is a strong indicator of embryo quality in human IVF. Hum Reprod. 2001; 16: 2652-7.

– Maheshwari A, Gibreel A, Siristatidis C, Bhattacharya S. Gonadotrophin-releasing hormone agonist protocols for pituitary suppression in assisted reproduction. Cochrane Database Syst Rev. 2011; 8: CD006919.

– Martikainen H, Orava M, Lakkakorpi J, Tuomivaara L. Day 2 elective single ET in clinical practice: better outcome in ICSI cycles. Hum Reprod. 2004; 19: 1364-6.

– Min JK, Breheny SA, MacLachlan V, Healy DL. What is the most relevant standard of success in assisted reproduction? The singleton, term gestation, live birth rate per cycle initiated: the BESST endpoint for assisted reproduction. Hum Reprod. 2004; 19: 3-7.

– Mortimer D. Sperm preparation methods. J Androl. 2000; 21: 357-66.

– Mulders A, Laven J, Imani B, Eijkemans M, Fauser B. IVF outcome in anovulatory infertility (WHO group 2) including PCOS-following previous unsuccessful ovulation induction. RBM Online. 2003; 7: 50-8.

– National Collaborating Centre for Women's and Children's Health. Factors affecting the outcome of IVF treatment. In: National Collaborating Centre for Women's and Children's Health, editors. Fertility assessment and treatment for people with fertility problems, 1st edition. RCOG press; 2004.

– Nyboe Andersen A, Goossens V, Gianaroli L, Felberbaum R, de Mouzon J, Nygren K. ART in Europe, 2003. Results generated from European registers by ESHRE. Hum Reprod. 2007; 22: 1513-25.

– Olson C, Keppler-Noreuil K, Romitti P, Budelier W, Ryan G, Sparks A, et al. IVF is associated with an increase in major birth defects. Fertil Steril. 2005; 84: 1308-15.

– Pandian Z, Gibreel A, Bhattacharya S. In vitro fertilisation for unexplained subfertility. Cochrane Database Syst Rev. 2015; 11: CD003357.

– Pandian Z, McTavish A, Aucott L, Hamilton M, Bhattacharya S. Interventions for 'poor responders' to controlled ovarian hyper stimulation (COH) in in-vitro fertilisation (IVF). Cochrane Database Syst Rev. 2010; 1: CD004379.

– Pasquali R, Gambineri A, Pagotto U. The impact of obesity on reproduction in women with PCOS. BJOG. 2006; 113: 1148-59.

– Pellestor F, Andreo B, Arnal F, Humeau C, Demaille J. Maternal aging and chromosomal abnormalities: new data drawn from in vitro unfertilized human oocytes. Hum Genet. 2003; 112: 195-203.

– Pinborg A, Loft A, Nyboe Andersen A. Neonatal outcome in a Danish national cohort of 8602 children born after IVF or ICSI: the role of twin pregnancy. Acta Obstet Gynecol Scand. 2004; 83: 1071-8.

– Practice Committee of the ASRM; Practice Committee of the SART. Preimplantation genetic testing: a Practice Committee opinion. Fertil Steril. 2008; 90: S136-43.

– Practice Committee of the ASRM; Practice Committee of the SART. Guidelines on number of ET. Fertil Steril. 2009; 92: 1518-9.

– Ragni G, Vegetti W, Riccaboni A, Engl B, Brigante C, Crosignani P. Comparison of GnRH agonists and antagonists in ART cycles of patients at high risk of OHSS. Hum Reprod. 2005; 20: 2421-5.

– Reefhuis J, Honein M, Schieve L, Correa A, Hobbs C, Rasmussen S; National Birth Defects Prevention Study. ART and major structural birth defects in the U.S. Hum Reprod. 2009; 24: 360-6.

– Revel A, Casper R. The use of LH-RH agonist to induce ovulation. In: Devroey P, editor. Infertility and Reproductive Medicine Clinics of North America. Philadelphia: WB Saunders; 2001: 105-18.

– Revised 2003 consensus on diagnostic criteria and long-term health risks related to PCOS. Hum Reprod. 2004; 19: 41-7.

– Rizk B, Aboulghar M. Classification, pathophysiology and management of OHSS. In: Brinsden P, editor. A Textbook of IVF and Assisted Reproduction, 2nd edition. Carnforth: Parthenon Publishing; 1999: 131-55.

– Rizk B, Nawar M. OHSS. In: Serhal P, Overton C, editors. Good Clinical Practice in Assisted Reproduction, 1st edition. Cambridge University Press; 2004: 146-66.

– Schieve L, Tatham L, Peterson H, Toner J, Jeng G. Spontaneous abortion among pregnancies conceived using ART in the U.S. Obstet Gynecol. 2003; 101: 959-67.

– Seif M, Edi-Osagie E, Farquhar C, Hooper L, Blake D, McGinlay P. Assisted hatching on assisted conception (IVF & ICSI). Cochrane Database Syst Rev. 2006; 1: CD001894.

– Serhal P, Overton C. OHSS. In: Rizk B, Nawar M, editors. Good Clinical Practice in Assisted Reproduction, 1st edition. Cambridge University Press; 2004.

– Sharlip I, Jarow J, Belker A, Lipshultz L, Sigman M, Thomas A, et al. Best practice policies for male infertility. Fertil Steril. 2002; 77: 873-82.

– Siristatidis C, Gibreel A, Basios G, Maheshwari A, Bhattacharya S. Gonadotrophin-releasing hormone agonist protocols for pituitary suppression in assisted reproduction. Cochrane Database Syst Rev. 2015; 11: CD006919.

– Siristatidis C, Maheshwari A, Vaidakis D, Bhattacharya S. In vitro maturation in subfertile women with polycystic ovarian syndrome undergoing assisted reproduction. Cochrane Database Syst Rev. 2018; 11: CD006606.

– Speroff L, Fritz M. Clinical Gynecological Endocrinolgy and Infertility, 7th edition. Philadelphia: Lippincott Williams and Wilkins; 2004: 1999-200.

– Steptoe P, Edwards R. Birth after reimplantation of a human embryo. Lancet. 1978; ii: 366.

– Sukuikkari AM. In-vitro maturation: Its role in fertility treatment. Curr Opin Obstet Gynecol. 2008; 20: 242-8.

– Tang H, Mourad S, Zhai S, Hart R. Dopamine agonists for preventing ovarian hyperstimulation syndrome. Cochrane Database Syst Rev. 2016; 11: CD008605.

– Tarlatzis B, Zepiridis L, Grimbizis G, Bontis J. Clinical management of low ovarian response to stimulation for IVF: a systematic review. Hum Reprod Update. 2003; 9: 61-76.

– Textbook of ARTs: Laboratory and clinical perspectives, 3rd edition. In: Gardner D, Weissman A, Howles C, Shoham Z, editors. 2009.

– The Practice Committee of the SART and the Practice Committee of the ASRM. Guidelines on number of embryos transferred. Fertil Steril. 2006; 86: S51-2.

– Tian L, Shen H, Lu Q, Norman R, Wang J. Insulin Resistance Increases the Risk of Spontaneous Abortion Following ART Treatment. J Clin Endocrinol Metab. 2007; 92: 1430-3.

– Tiitinen A, Halttunen M, Harkki P, Vuoristo P, Hyden-Granskog C. Elective single ET: the value of cryopreservation. Hum Reprod. 2001; 16: 1140-4.

– Tummon I, Gavrilova-Jordan L, Allemand M, Session D. Polycystic ovaries and OHSS: a systematic review. Acta Obstet Gynecol Scand. 2005; 84: 611-6.

– van der Linden M, Buckingham K, Farquhar C, Kremer J, Metwally M. Luteal phase support for assisted reproduction cycles. Cochrane Database Syst Rev. 2011; 10: CD009154.

– Veeck L. An Atlas of Human Gametes and Conceptuses. New York, NY: The Pathenon Publishing Group; 1999.

– Wang J, Davies M, Norman R. Body mass and probability of pregnancy during assisted reproduction treatment: retrospective study. BMJ. 2000; 321: 1320-1

– Wang J, Davies M, Norman R. PCOS and the risk of spontaneous abortion following ART treatment. Hum Reprod. 2001; 16: 2606-9.

– Wang Y, Sullivan E, Black D, Dean J, Bryant J, Chapman M. Preterm birth and low birth weight after ART-related pregnancy in Australia between 1996 and 2000. Fertil Steril. 2005; 83: 1650-8.

– Whelan JG 3rd, Vlahos N. The OHSS. Fertil Steril. 2000; 73: 883-96.

– Wong K, van Wely , Mol F, Repping S, Mastenbroek S. Fresh versus frozen embryo transfers in assisted reproduction. Cochrane Database Syst Rev. 2017; 3: CD011184.

– Wongtra-Ngan S, Vutyavanich T, Brown J. Follicular flushing during oocyte retrieval in ARTs. Cochrane Database Syst Rev. 2010; 9: CD004634.

− Wright VC, Chang J, Jeng G, Macaluso M. ART surveillance - U.S., 2003. MMWR Surveill Summ. 2006; 55: 1-22.

− Youssef M, Mourad S. Volume expanders for the prevention of ovarian hyperstimulation syndrome. Cochrane Database Syst Rev. 2016; 8: CD001302.

− Zegers-Hochschild F, Adamson G, de Mouzon J, Ishihara O, Mansour R, Sullivan E, et al. International Committee for Monitoring ART (ICMART) and the WHO revised glossary of ART terminology, 2009. Fertil Steril. 2009; 92: 1520-24.

www.ingramcontent.com/pod-product-compliance
Lightning Source LLC
Chambersburg PA
CBHW030658220526

45463CB00005B/1823